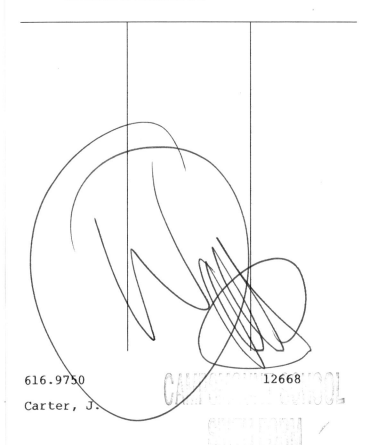

The allergy exclusion diet: the 28-day
plan to solve your food intolerances

CAMPSMOUNT SCHOOL

the Allergy Exclusion Diet

The 28-day plan to solve your food intolerances

JILL CARTER AND ALISON EDWARDS

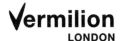

Vermilion
LONDON

First published in 2002 by Vermilion,
an imprint of Ebury Press, Random House,
20 Vauxhall Bridge Road, London SW1V 2SA
www.randomhouse.co.uk

Random House Australia (Pty) Limited
20 Alfred Street, Milsons Point, Sydney,
New South Wales 2061, Australia

Random House New Zealand Limited
18 Poland Road, Glenfield,
Auckland 10, New Zealand

Random House South Africa (Pty) Limited
Endulini, 5a Jubilee Road,
Parktown 2193, South Africa

The Random House Group Limited Reg. No. 954009

Papers used by Vermilion are natural, recyclable
products made from wood grown in sustainable forests.

Designed by Lovelock & Co.

Printed and bound in Great Britain
by Mackays of Chatham plc, Chatham, Kent

A CIP catalogue record for this book is available from the British Library.

ISBN 0 09 188221 4

A note to the reader

The information contained in this book is given for the purposes of helping people who suspect they may have a food allergy or intolerance. Before following the advice, the reader is advised to give careful consideration to the nature of their problem and to consult a health care practitioner if in any doubt. This is particularly important for dealing with babies and young children, and in cases of diabetes, severe depression and schizophrenia. This book should not be used as a substitute for medical treatment and whilst every care has been taken to ensure the accuracy of the information, the authors and publishers cannot accept any responsibility for any problems arising out of experimentation with the method described.

contents

introduction

Poised on the threshold of change, your mind whirls around those favourite foods you love and crave – the chocolates, the pizzas, the ice creams and the take-aways. Could there really be some 'hidden enemy' lurking in such delicacies? Could just a simple food allergy to these have been spoiling your life all these years? Could you reduce your dependency on painkillers, antacids and all those other palliative medicines, just by altering your diet?

The answer quite simply is yes. This book will first explain how food allergies can affect you and secondly will show you how to alleviate them. It will then guide you through the Elimination Diet, giving you recipes for each meal. This will enable you to discover the hidden culprits that are preventing you from feeling really well.

If you are already allergic or intolerant to certain foods you will probably become allergic to others because if a food is eaten too frequently, the body is unable to break it down and process it completely. It can therefore become overloaded. Even if you don't suffer

Case study

Jack, aged six, was constantly bothered by weeping eczema. Twice he was admitted to hospital as a toddler and on one occasion he had scratched himself so badly that he had to be sedated. Then his mother discovered he was intolerant to all dairy produce and all pulses. Almost overnight he started to improve. For the first time since he was born he started to sleep through the night, his yellow sores disappeared and he became a different child.

from allergies, it is likely that you will feel the effects of the overload. This is where the Rotation Diet, which follows the Elimination Diet, comes in.

A rotation diet offers a way of spacing foods so you can recover from the effects of a food before it is eaten again. It was originally designed to help people who are allergic to foods but it can be wonderfully beneficial for everyone. Many people with highly demanding lifestyles find that their energy levels increase and they feel much better when they rotate their foods. After all, it was not so long ago that we depended on food grown close at hand, and the seasons of the year dictated a natural rotation.

If you have discovered that you are allergic to certain foods, either from following the Elimination Diet or from the many tests available, it is important that you should understand how to plan and use a rotation diet. However, the prospect of embarking on a rotation diet can be so daunting that all but the most determined have either given up in the early stages or not started at all. This book will give you a clear understanding of the principles and show you just how to follow them. Once grasped, the diet can then be adapted to your individual needs. With delicious and nourishing recipes for you to experiment with and enjoy, this book will give you the chance to sample foods that you may never have thought to try before.

There is good news for weight-watchers too. Eliminating food

Daphne (8 years old) was constantly away from school due to persistent headaches, diarrhoea and tummy aches. She was referred to her local hospital and after counselling treatment failed, she was referred to a dietician who put her on a milk, egg, beef and poultry-free diet. When this did not help, she was advised to stop all preservatives. Her mother then found a natural medicine centre and a test revealed reactions to wheat, oats, barley and rye. Because there had been a long history of illness a rotation diet was recommended. Milk, eggs, beef and poultry were returned to the diet in the rotation but the cereal grains were strictly avoided. Her mother wrote a report stating 'no headaches and tummy aches; no time away from school; she attended willingly and happily every day and her general complexion is now pink and healthy rather than the black eyes and a white face. She has had no diarrhoea for eight weeks'.

allergies and then following the Rotation Diet could be the critical move needed to lose those extra pounds or, if you are underweight, to establishing your ideal weight.

If you have been a migraine, eczema or asthma sufferer for years; if you are experiencing pain and stiffness creeping into muscles and joints; if you have digestive problems or if you suffer from depression, mood changes and fatigue; if you have sinus problems, earache, tinnitus or permanent catarrh; if you are concerned because your child is overactive and unable to sleep, or if you have any of the symptoms listed in the next chapter, then this book could be the answer for you and a major step towards enhancing not only your own health but also the health of others around you.

the allergy exclusion diet

chapter 1
an understanding
of allergies

It is useful to understand exactly what allergies are, the way they can affect you and their possible causes. The word 'allergy' has become a catchword, particularly in connection with food. What we are usually talking about, though, is a food intolerance rather than an allergy.

If you were to have a 'true' allergic reaction to a food, you would know about it immediately as the initial response can be very dramatic. With this type of abnormal hypersensitivity, your body's defence mechanisms would be alerted. Hives, rashes and puffy eyes could appear within seconds, an asthmatic attack, swelling of joints, vomiting and nausea could then follow and, in some severe cases, an anaphylactic shock or an apparent heart attack. Classic foods that cause this type of reaction are shellfish, strawberries, cashew nuts and peanuts. If you are allergic to something, a reaction will occur each time the particular food is eaten. The condition is well recognised by doctors and laboratory tests can confirm the culprits. The problem is then overcome simply by avoiding the offending food.

The words 'intolerance' and 'sensitivity' are both used to describe the other type of allergy, of which orthodox medicine now recognises the existence. According to the Royal College of Physicians and the British Nutritional Foundation, 'an intolerance is a reaction caused by a food but the mechanism is not clear'. It seems that an intolerance, like an allergy, may also result from a misdirected response of the body's immune system but the reactions are less apparent. The immune system, which is designed to protect your body from invading organisms such as bacteria and viruses, makes antibodies, which kill or neutralise the invaders. In people with allergies, however, the antibodies attack normally harmless substances such as food. This is when a reaction occurs. As you continue to eat the substance, though, perhaps even two or three times a day, your body will endeavour to adapt. Your reactions will become reduced and the symptoms masked, therefore presenting a far more vague and complex picture, so much so that you may have difficulty associating these symptoms with the foods you are eating.

You will often crave and become addicted to the particular food to which you are intolerant. You can give up anything else, you may say, but not my morning cup of coffee, glass of wine or buttered toast. You may not consciously realise your craving but will be regularly topping yourself up with the particular food to satisfy your yearnings. This is because you will usually experience a 'lift' after eating a food to which you are intolerant as your body will be producing large amounts of adrenaline to fight the reaction. However, the beneficial feeling will then disappear after one or two hours. As time goes by, and your body starts to get tired from so much over-stimulation, you will need more and more of the food to feel 'good'. In extreme cases, this process is similar to drug, alcohol and cigarette addiction.

If you continue to subject your body to the food for long enough, you can reach a stage of exhaustion. Collapsing over your desk at work, suffering 'burn out' before your years, or simply cutting short your trip around the shops; these are all signs that your body's defence mechanism can no longer cope.

The causes of allergies and food intolerances

Allergies and food intolerances are on the increase. This may be due to a number of factors of which pollution is one. Today, man is exposed to more chemicals than ever before; in the air we breathe, in the chemically contaminated food, water and prescription medicines we ingest and from the many toxic substances that our skin comes into contact with. Our daily diet contains pesticides, mycotoxins, dyes, additives and many other chemicals. In addition, heavy metals such as lead from petrol fumes and mercury from amalgam tooth fillings can overload the natural detoxifying pathways of the body, particularly in the liver. The result is that the defence systems of the body become over-worked and over-extended and so, not surprisingly, fail to work efficiently.

Nutritional deficiency can also play a part. The increasing use of chemicals in farming as well as the transport, processing and storage of foods for long periods can all lead to the decrease of valuable vitamins and minerals in foods. These vitamins and minerals are vital for a strong immune system, and since there is a noticeable correlation between immune deficiency and allergies, it is probable that if you have allergies or intolerances, you will be deficient in many vitamins and minerals. This is particularly likely if you eat a lot of refined sugar, milk and wheat since these foods can deplete your vitamin and mineral levels. Approximately 48 per cent of the raw molasses extracted from sugar cane consists of vitamins and minerals that are necessary for the body to break down and metabolise the sugar molecules. However, most people eat white processed sugar, which has none of these nutrients left, so eating this will actually draw on the body's reserves of minerals and vitamins. Wheat, which is high in gluten, a sticky, gluey-like substance, can coat the lining of the intestines and therefore prevent the proper absorption of nutrients from the diet. Similarly, milk can damage the lining of the intestines.

Sugar and wheat can also encourage an overgrowth of unfriendly micro-organisms such as candida albicans in the gut. Candida is a yeast growth present in and on most people. It is normally controlled by the immune defences and the 'friendly flora' in the intestines. When the immune system has been weakened, for example by a chronic viral infection such as glandular fever, or the internal flora has been depleted, perhaps by antibiotics or contraceptive pills, the candida can grow out of control and the condition called candidiasis manifests. This condition effects the mucus membranes and allows undigested food particles to pass through the walls of the intestines and trigger food intolerances. Parasites such as Giardia Lamblia, may also trigger food intolerances in the same way by damaging the intestines and destroying the friendly bacteria.

Another contributory factor to allergies and food intolerances may be bottle-feeding with cow's milk. An infant's intestinal tract is very porous and it takes between six to twelve months before it can screen out the large molecules in substances such as wheat, milk products, fish and egg white. So, if a baby is fed on cow's milk or solid food during the early months, its digestive system may not be able to cope. In addition, it will be missing the protective substances in the mother's milk and colostrum, so it will not be able to build up a healthy immune system.

There could also be a possible hereditary cause. Parents with allergies and food intolerances tend to give birth to children with allergies and intolerances but whether this is passed on through the genes or the placenta via the blood, is not known.

Stress can increase allergies and food intolerances. People who feel stressed, look for reasons causing the stress and may blame it entirely on their relationships or the work environment. When the diet is altered, frequently stress decreases considerably. Quite often when you feel stressed you should think about your diet rather than look for the things in your life that cause you stress.

Certain foods can exacerbate stress. Caffeine, for example, can cause anxiety, palpitations, irritability and insomnia, and food additives have been proved to cause hyperactivity. Quite often when you feel stressed you should think about your diet rather than look for the things in your life that cause you stress.

In the past, germs have determined the pattern of illness in our society. Today, this is still true but we have entered an era of man-made illness in which allergies and food intolerances are increasingly prevalent.

The symptoms of a food intolerance

All manner of symptoms may be the result of a food intolerance, ranging from headaches and migraine, chronic fatigue, fluctuating weight, digestive problems, pains in the neck, joints and muscles, arthritis, asthma, eczema, poor concentration and dizziness, to mood swings, emotional outbursts and even violent behaviour (see also chart on page 14). In addition it has been found that food intolerances can be one of the causes of many chronic conditions such as ME, AIDS and cancer, due to the depletion of the immune system.

The symptoms can also change. An elderly woman suffering from arthritis, for example, may have had constant feeding problems, windy colicky pains, constipation and teething troubles in early childhood. She may have suffered from eczema, hayfever, catarrh, repeated coughs, colds and ear infections, and was perhaps hyperactive and had learning and co-ordination difficulties at school. Later on in her life, she may have suffered from migraines, headaches, asthma, acne and depression. She may also have been affected by hormonal changes, particularly at puberty, during pregnancy, postnatally or during the menopause. This would have given rise to PMT, heavy or irregular periods, early morning sickness during pregnancy and postnatal and menopausal depression.

Of course, some of the symptoms listed on page 14 may be due to other reasons. Insomnia, for example, could be due to a specific incident, which is causing you stress, or backache due to poor seating at work. But if you are experiencing many of these symptoms frequently and severely, and not always for any apparent reason, you will probably find that allergies and/or intolerances are the cause. So take note if you have inexplicable panic attacks, for example, or if you feel irritable for no reason or have any other persistent problem. For by discovering your allergies and/or intolerances, you may discover the reason for such symptoms.

Symptoms that indicate a food intolerance

- Overweight, underweight, fluctuating weight.
- Itching or burning skin, eczema, urticaria, dandruff, acne, varicose veins.
- Cramps, nausea, vomiting, diarrhoea, constipation, bloating, flatulence, colitis, ulcerative colitis, irritable bowel, colic, indigestion, anaemia.
- Discomfort in the muscles of the neck.
- Backache, aching muscles or joints, fibrositis, arthritis, tingling in the muscles.
- Insomnia, waking in the night, poor sleep pattern.
- Impaired energy, chronic fatigue.
- Weeping/itching eyes, visual problems, sensitivity to bright lights.
- Sneezing, sinusitis, runny nose, polyps, post-nasal drip, hay fever, nose bleeds.
- Ringing in the ears, earache.
- Sore throat, hoarseness, cough, catarrh, asthma, wheezing, bronchitis, breathlessness.
- Cold/hot sweating extremities, chilblains, hot flushes.
- Fast/slow pulse, high/low blood pressure, palpitations, unexplained anginal pain.
- Dark puffy circles under eyes, constant bruising.
- Painful irregular periods, PMT, thrush.
- Frequent urination, bed wetting, water retention, cystitis, frequent colds or infections, excessive sweating, low blood sugar.
- Inexplicable fatigue, sleepiness, drowsiness after meals, waking up tired, sleep walking, nightmares, hallucinations.
- Persistent tension/anxiety/nervousness, panic attacks, poor tolerance to pain.
- Headaches, migraine, convulsions, blackouts, vertigo, dizzy spells, poor co-ordination.
- Mental confusion, poor concentration, forgetfulness, depression, blank mind, difficulty in making decisions.

- Hyperactivity, irritability, aggressiveness, violence.
- Delayed crawling/walking/talking, learning disabilities.
- Colic, fretfulness, earache, croup.
- Inability to delay or miss a meal, obsessional eating, craving a special food, constant snacking, poor appetite.
- Feeling unwell when food or drink are missed.
- Feeling immediately better after obtaining the food to which sensitive.
- Tender gums, bleeding gums, mouth ulcers, cracks in lips, sore tongue.
- White marks on your nails, splitting nails, stria on your skin, dry flaky skin, pale in colour.
- Excessive hair loss, prematurely grey hair.
- Little desire for sex.
- Infertility.

Detecting allergies and food intolerances

Detecting allergies and food intolerances can be complicated but if you follow the Elimination Diet given in this book you should find most, if not all, of the answers. Alternatively, you could have your allergies or food intolerances tested at a natural health clinic. In this case it is worth bearing in mind, that 'allergy tests' are not always accurate and that allergies and intolerances can anyway change or increase. A period of general ill-health, a virus infection or any increased stress in your life can lead to an increase of allergic responses. Furthermore, assessing your own problems will give you more control over your body. So you may decide that you want to follow the Elimination Diet before embarking on the Rotation Diet.

chapter 2
preparing for
your diet

The diets in this book cannot be followed half-heartedly. If they are to be successful, it is important to take time to plan and prepare. You need time to collect the new foods you are going to use and to find shops to supply you.

Choose a quiet time of the year to embark on your diet, away from Christmas, festive occasions or anniversaries when it could be difficult to stick to your regime. For the week prior to starting and during the time you are on either of the diets, you will need to keep a food diary. Make a list on the left of the page of everything that passes your lips, including drinks and snacks. On the right-hand side, write down any reactions or feelings you experience and record on a scale of 1 to 10 the severity of these reactions.

On starting, it is very important not to include anything else in your diet. Alcohol, coffee, strong tea, cocoa, cola, chocolate, spices or other stimulants, including tobacco, increase any adverse response that may be occurring. This is particularly important when following the Elimination Diet.

This may seem difficult and time consuming. However, the benefits to your health and to your life will far exceed any minor difficulties you may encounter. As long as you take the time to buy the right foods and to cook them correctly, you will be able to manage these diets easily. In addition, the recipes have been designed so you can take any meals with you, if you need to. For example, if you work full-time you can easily make your lunch either the night before or in the morning and then take it with you to work. The same goes for picnics, travelling, or any other occasions when you cannot eat at home.

Reactions

It is important, to prepare yourself for any possible reactions, especially at the beginning. Do make sure you start either diet when you can devote time and energy to it, rather than when you are very busy with other things. And be prepared to take it easy if you need to.

Withdrawal symptoms

When you first start either of the diets, withdrawal symptoms are likely to occur and are usually a sign that the diet is working. These may take the form of headaches, blurred vision, nausea, an infection, feelings similar to a hangover or simply an increase in the symptoms you are trying to reduce. These symptoms can last for four or five days, after which time they usually cease and a marked improvement in health is observed. In the case of long-standing illness, though, you may have to wait longer. Psychologically, you may feel uneasy, depressed, lack zest and be quite bad tempered. Know that this is natural and that the body is just allowing you to have a last look at what has been suppressed, smothered and unacknowledged in the past and is now clearing. Know too, that these feelings are only temporary; do not see them as bad but just accept them, be 'still' and allow yourself to feel them. You will be amazed how quickly they will then disappear. Having a glass of water, doing some deep breathing or going for a walk can also help.

You will also find that you will 'react' if you eat something to which you are allergic or intolerant. Again, reactions vary from person to person and can even vary for each particular person.

Different foods, for example, may produce different reactions and different circumstances, such as stress or pollution can also effect the reactions. It is worth noting the reactions, particularly as the 'clearer' your body becomes, the more noticeable the reactions will be. One fail-safe way of discovering whether or not you are allergic or intolerant to something is by testing your pulse. If it has quickened, then your body is reacting.

The pulse test

Before eating a food, rest for a while and take your pulse. Count the beats of your heart by lightly placing your fingers on the artery on the underside of your wrist on the side of your thumb, for one minute. Then remain resting and take your pulse 15 minutes and 30 minutes after eating. If your pulse rate increases by 8 beats or more you are probably reacting to a food.

To ease symptoms

- Take 1 tsp of bicarbonate of soda and ½ tsp of potassium bicarbonate dissolved in a glass of water. Potassium bicarbonate is not so easily obtainable but some chemists may be able to supply you. Capsules of bicarbonate of soda mixed with potassium in the correct proportions can be purchased and may be useful when away from home.
- A herbal alternative is meadowsweet. An infusion can be made by steeping 25 g of herb in 500 ml of boiling water. Strain and use in doses of 75 ml.
- Vitamin C can also be very effective (take 1-2 g with a glass of water) as can drinking plenty of water, which will help flush the system.

Removing chemicals

If you have not experienced any withdrawal symptoms and your symptoms are still occurring, or are only slightly reduced, it may be that you are reacting to an environmental substance. If you put all chemical substances from your home in a garage or shed and then find you feel much better, you can then work out which substances are causing the problems. You may think this sounds a bit extreme but it is usually well worth the effort. Examples of these are strong smelling or highly perfumed products such as dry cleaning fumes, harsh detergents, biological washing powders, fabric conditioners, shoe polish, household cleaning products such as artificial air fresheners, cosmetic aerosols and sprays, e.g. deodorants, hair sprays and perfume.

Bars of pure soap and soap flakes are good alternatives for washing clothes and domestic borax, soda crystals or vinegar and water for household cleaning. Sodium bicarbonate can be used as a deodorant and pure alcohol instead of aftershave lotion. Simple wax and liquid polishes which do not smell can be used instead of solid wax shoe polish. Most water-based paints are safe but new carpets, furniture, paint, floor waxes and sealants can cause problems, as can air conditioning, gas, oil and paraffin. Be wary of foam-backed carpets and vinyl wallpapers, car fumes and gas. It is also important, of course, to avoid smoking, alcohol, unnecessary

Case study

Illness plagued **Karin** from birth. During her early years she was constantly troubled by colds, earache and sleepless nights. Her speech development was delayed and it was difficult to understand her until she was nearly seven years old. Dyslexic problems were diagnosed and several years extra help at school were required. She then became asthmatic at the age of eight. It was then that she was put on a wheat-free diet. The asthmatic attacks ceased, and no medication was required. Now, twenty years on she has never had any further symptoms of asthma. The dyslexia problems were more difficult to solve though, and these persisted throughout her school years. Eventually, however, she discovered that she was reacting to numerous foods, chemicals, gas and other fumes. Having discovered the cause of her dyslexia, she was able to take steps to avoid the environmental substances. She then rapidly took some exams and entered a university. She gained a first class honours degree.

medications or recreational drugs. Toothpaste is another item to be careful of; sugar-free types are now widely available.

General guidelines for making the most of the diets

- Good planning can help to pave the way to managing your diets successfully. It is helpful to look ahead and stock your larder with the basic grain cereals, dried beans, lentils, etc. A list of the most useful foods to keep in stock is given on page 23. Always have some of your good 'safe' foods on hand so if you do start reacting to any particular item, there is something to fall back on.

- If you buy anything that is packaged, you need to take great care to study the labels. It is worth noting, however, that in the UK, labels do not have to declare substances where the content is less than 1 per cent. Packets and tins of convenience food can therefore frequently contain wheat or other grains, potato flour, milk powder, egg and sugar without you knowing. The list at the back of the book may help you.

- Avoid buying unwrapped fruit and vegetables exposed to street traffic fumes and wash all fruit and vegetables thoroughly, discarding the outer leaves of lettuce, cabbage, etc. You can use 500 mg Vitamin C powder, or 1 tbsp vinegar to 1 litre of water, to help remove heavy metals and pesticide residues.

- Drink plenty of mineral water, between meals, 3 to 4 litres a day. It is best to buy the water in glass bottles but if you do have to resort to plastic bottles, never leave them in the sun or around in hot weather when the chemicals in the plastic could leach into the water. Do not drink straight from the bottle unless you are going to use the whole bottle within a short space of time. The microbes from your mouth can breed quickly.

- Your usual prescription medicines can be taken but try to decrease tablets like tranquillisers and sleeping tablets and avoid all unnecessary tablets. Also avoid all vitamins and minerals as they contain fillers and other hidden substances that could interfere with the diet. If any of your prescription tablets are sugar coated, you can wash the sugar off.

▧ Choose long or short grain, organically grown wholemeal rice, obtainable from health food stores or some supermarkets. The rice should be rinsed thoroughly before using and you may want to soak the rice in mineral water for 6 to 8 hours prior to cooking. This brings it 'alive' and makes it more nutritious.

▧ Use green, brown or puy lentils but as red lentils have been processed these will not sprout. They are only good

The soaking and sprouting of beans, grains and seeds

Alfalfa, linseeds, fenugreek, sesame, pumpkin, sunflower and oats will need at least 6 hours soaking time. Beans, almonds and other nuts, wheat, rice, millet and rye will need at least twelve hours.

Special bean sprouters may be purchased for this purpose but using a jam jar can be just as simple and effective.

1 Take a handful of beans, wash thoroughly and place in a jam jar. Cover with about three times as much water. Place a piece of muslin or screen over the top for draining and leave to soak overnight.

2 Rinse and drain through the muslin top and place the jar, on its side, in a dark, airy cupboard. Repeat this twice a day for 3 to 5 days.

3 On the last 2 days, place the jar in the sunlight, keeping them moist while they grow green with chlorophyll.

Refrigerate in a covered container and use raw in salads, soups, etc. It is advantageous to sprout all beans for 2 to 3 days prior to cooking. Many people who may have difficulty digesting beans will find them acceptable when prepared in this way.

for very young children or anyone who is unable to cope with the high fibre content in sprouted lentils. Sprouting greatly enhances the nutrient value and digestibility of these foods. Many beans, grains, seeds and even some nuts will sprout. When water is added, many of the enzyme and metabolic inhibitors that are designed to keep the seed from germinating until the allotted time, are washed out. If ingested, these can block our absorption of calcium, zinc and other minerals. The water also activates the germination process and starts the pre-digestion of the proteins, fats and carbohydrates into amino acids, fatty acids and simple carbohydrates respectively. The synthesis of many vitamins also takes place including Vitamin B-complex, C and E, and these, together with the mineral content, increase immensely.

- The best way to cook vegetables is to steam or boil them in a little water. Any leftover water can be used as stock or simply drunk as it will contain many of the nutrients.
- Avoid all foods containing additives, preservatives and colourings including margarines. Although we need to have plenty of poly-unsaturated oil in our diet, margarines are not a good source.
- Poly-unsaturated oils contain fatty acids that are essential for health but these can only be found in certain unrefined and cold pressed oils as the refining process can turn the fatty acids into harmful trans-fatty acids. Oils should be purchased in glass bottles and refrigerated once opened as any oil or fat can become rancid when exposed to light or air for any length of time.
- Take great care when cooking with oil. Both fats and oils can produce very toxic substances if over-heated or if exposed to light or air for any length of time. This is why lower temperatures have been used in the recipes. Butter or ghee, pure lard (organic), tropical fats (coconut, palm kernel), sesame and olive oil in this order, produce the least

amount of toxic substances when heated. If you do need to fry, you can cool-fry, by putting a little water into the pan with the fat or oil. When using a wok, use a little water rather than oil.

- Check sell-buy labels and avoid all sauces and composite foods, e.g. sausages, burgers, etc.
- Do also allow your diet to be as varied as possible. The wealth of whole foods available mean that you can eat delicious, exciting meals without having to smother the food in additive-filled sauces. Instead you will find that you soon begin to appreciate the more subtle and natural flavours of the foods instead.
- Whenever possible, sit down and eat in a peaceful and settled atmosphere and give mindful attention to the food you are eating. 'Energy flows where attention goes', so your digestion and appreciation of the food will be greatly enhanced if you do this. Try to chew well and avoid reading newspapers over a meal, watching television, eating on the run or anything else that causes stress on the body.
- Most of the recipes in this book are designed for four people, as this is the average family size. Even though only one member of the family may be following the diet, it will be of great help to that person if the rest of the family eats the same meal, all of whom will benefit.
- Most importantly, work with a good will, love and care when preparing and cooking food. The best food can be marred and ruined for everyone if prepared in a hectic or negative frame of mind.

Some of the foods you may want to buy for your larder

Agar agar This is a seaweed-based setting agent similar to gelatine. It is rich in protein and calcium and is easy to digest. It may be bought as granules or flakes. The granules are more processed but stronger. To make, use 1 tsp granules to 250 ml of liquid. With the flakes, use 1 tbsp to 250 ml of liquid. For both types, mix the agar agar with some or all of the liquid, bring to the boil and simmer for one minute. It sets quickly but may be re-heated to liquefy without spoiling.

Amaranth

A relatively new cereal to our stores and useful for highly sensitive people who are unlikely to have built up an intolerance to it. It is gluten free and contains all of the eight amino acids and is also rich in iron. It is similar to millet in appearance and can be cooked in the same way. Due to its comparatively high protein content, it is also a useful food for vegans who are intolerant to nuts.

Barley

The major grain used in the manufacture of alcohol. It is a glutinous cereal and can be bought as a flour, flakes, as pearl barley or pot barley. As pearl barley has been processed, it will not sprout so it is better to buy pot barley.

Buckwheat

A gluten- and wheat-free seed that can be cooked and treated like rice. It is rich in potassium and the amino acid, lysine, which most grains lack. It also contains rutin, which is good for strengthening the blood capillaries, helps improve circulation and stabilises blood pressure.

Dairy foods

Allergies and intolerances to cow's milk products are extremely common but the protein in goat's and sheep's milk is more easily digested. Live yoghurt, preferably sheep's or goat's, and some cheeses in which the milk has been partially broken down by enzyme action are often tolerated more easily by many. Both goat's and sheep's milk will freeze, although goat's milk can have a somewhat 'goaty' flavour unless it is very fresh. Clarified butter can often be tolerated by milk-sensitive people. This is because the milk protein has been separated. It can be bought as 'ghee' at Indian food shops and at most supermarkets or can be

the allergy exclusion diet

made at home. To make, melt a pack of butter over gentle heat, allow to cook slightly and then pour off carefully into a glass jar. The proteins in the butter will have settled on the bottom of the pan. Ghee and butter are the most stable fats for use in cooking.

Flax seed oil (linseed oil)

One of the richest and most stable sources of omega 3 fatty acids. Use on salads or take by the spoonful, 1–2 tbsp a day, but it is not suitable for cooking.

Hemp seed/oil

Hemp is one of the sturdiest and fastest growing plants on the planet and a plant well favoured by environmentalists. Its long penetrating roots draw minerals buried deep in the soil up to the surface, enriching the soil on which it grows and requiring no pesticides, herbicides and little fertilizer. Hemp seeds are rich in magnesium, potassium, sulphur and other key elements and contain all the essential amino acids in an easily digestible form. They contain the richest known source of essential fatty acids in their oil and in the perfect ratio for human nutritional needs. The drug, tetrahydracannabinol is contained in the leaves and the flowers of certain strains of the hemp plant and it is for this reason that growing hemp is illegal. However, the drug is not present in the seeds, which are legal and obtainable. They are best eaten raw or ground and made into butters. They can be also added to flours to make hemp breads etc.

Kamut

An ancient, non-hybridised grain, now being produced in the United States and slowly coming on to the market in Great Britain that many 'wheat allergic' people can tolerate. It is a variety of high-protein, low-gluten wheat with kernels two to three times the size of wheat grains. Because of its low gluten content, though, it is not so good for making bread.

Kelp

A natural seaweed product that is extremely high in minerals and trace elements, particularly iodine. It may be used as a substitute for salt.

Millet
Gluten-free but cheaper to buy than the other grains mentioned and obtainable at most stores. It is the most alkaline of the grains and contains all but one of the essential amino acids. It also contains potassium, iron and magnesium and is an excellent source of silicon, which is a mineral essential for healthy bones, teeth, nails and hair. Millet is particularly good for the health and function of the stomach, spleen and pancreas. Cook as for rice, using 1 cup of millet to 2 cups of water and cook for 25 minutes.

Miso
A Japanese seasoning paste similar to yeast extracts in taste and colour. It is made from fermented rice, barley or soya beans so check the labelling carefully when buying. It is an excellent source of nutrients and is useful as a flavouring for soups and stews.

Olive oil
Rich in mono-unsaturates, though low in essential fatty acids and the cold pressed, virgin olive oil is the only unrefined oil sold on the mass market. Due to its relative stability and to the ease with which it can be extracted, i.e. it does not require high pressure pressing equipment, many of its health-giving properties remain intact. It contains vitamin E, phytosterols, chlorophyll, magnesium, carotene and other beneficial minor ingredients, unique to olives. Use virgin olive oil on salads, stirring into vegetables and soups and for low temperature cooking as well.

Pepper
Black and white pepper can be used on cold or warm food. However, it is important not to heat it or add it to very hot food as it then becomes an irritant to the intestinal mucosa.

Pulses (dried peas, beans and lentils)
These are a good source of protein and fibre. When mixed with a grain such as rice, they provide a complete protein meal, i.e. one that contains all the essential amino acids. It is recommended that these are sprouted for 2 to 3 days prior to cooking or for 3 to 5 days for eating raw as this will increase their nutrient value greatly, enhance their digestibility and reduce cooking time.

the allergy exclusion diet

Quinoa Can be used in the same way as millet. It contains all eight essential amino acids and is extremely rich in calcium and iron. It can be cooked in the granule form or the seeds can be ground to a flour in a liquidiser or coffee grinder.

Rice One of the oldest cultivated grains. Generally speaking, it is a safe food for most people but for those who have used it as a staple food for many years may need to check carefully for any intolerance. Choose organically grown, short or long grain varieties. Wholegrain, basmati, wild and wholegrain noodles are also available in health food stores. Vermicelli (white Chinese noodles) may be useful in some recipes. Always wash rice grains before cooking. Soaking for 6 to 8 hours prior to cooking will 'bring the rice alive' and reduce cooking time.

Safflower, soya bean and sunflower seed oil These oils are highly nutritious and rich in poly-unsaturates and essential fatty acids but only when unrefined and cold pressed. Use in salads and add to soups and vegetables when off the boil. If you do need to use these oils in baking, keep the temperature of the oven to below 160°C.

Sesame seed oil Should be unrefined, untoasted and cold pressed. In this state it is a rich source of omega 6 essential fatty acids. Use cold, sprinkled on salads. It remains reasonably stable when heated so it can be used for low temperature cooking.

Sorghum An African grain, now grown in many other parts of the world. It is similar in composition to corn but higher in protein and is available at some health food stores or by mail order.

Spelt flour An ancient precursor of modern day wheat, usually grown organically and is often more easily tolerated.

Sweet potatoes, yams, eddoes and dasheen
Available in most large supermarkets and are sold at many West

Indian food stores. They are all high in carbohydrates and may be used like potatoes. It is also possible to buy sweet potato and yam flours. The flesh of the sweet potato is either whitish or orange and due to its sweet flavour, can be used in sweet or savory cooking.

Tahini A nut butter made from roasted ground sesame seeds and oil and used as a spread, topping, in dips and dressings, sauces and soups.

Tamari A naturally produced, wheat-free soya sauce.

Tempeh Cultured from cooked, split soya beans in a similar way to cheese.

Tofu A high protein, low fat curd made from soya milk. Both tofu and tempeh are very digestible.

Tropical oils Unrefined and cold pressed palm oil or coconut oil are much more stable when heated than any of the poly-unsaturated oils and are therefore more suitable for cooking purposes. If you are able to obtain these, you can use them instead of sunflower and safflower oils, in the baking recipes.

Umeboshi plums Japanese plums that have been picked green and pickled in brine with shiso (perilla) leaves which give them the pink colour. They are rich in enzymes and are a good digestive aid. They may be bought at health food shops, whole and also as a purée.

Walnut oil An excellent source of omega 6 and a smaller amount of omega 3 essential fatty acids as long as it is unrefined and cold pressed.

Wheat Contains gluten, but when the grains are sprouted, the gluten and gluten-like substances found in rye, barley and oats are broken down by the enzyme action. You may therefore find you can tolerate wheat and similarly, rye, barley and oats when they are sprouted. In addition, some people find that they can tolerate durum wheat found in wheat pasta, couscous, bulgur wheat and semolina more easily than the strong wheat flour used in baking. Bread made with French flour may also be an alternative. Wheat seems to absorb more of the pesticides and artificial fertilisers used in farming than other grains, so it is important to buy organically grown wheat.

Wheat germ oil One of the richest sources of Vitamin E and may also protect the heart and help nerve regeneration. Many people, intolerant to the wheat grain, find they can tolerate wheat germ oil. Take by the spoonful or cold, on salads.

Choose foods that are natural, whole, pure and unprocessed, buy organic produce and meat from animals which have been reared in humane conditions, wherever possible. This will reduce the amount of drugs and chemicals you are ingesting.

Adapting the diets to your needs

By following the diets in this book you will be restricting what you eat for several months. During this time you may want to alter the diets and you will also need to consider what to do when away from home, eating out in restaurants, with friends or when travelling.

Case study

Patricia, aged 35 years, heard she could lose weight by avoiding certain foods. Following a test for food intolerances she was advised to avoid wheat and sugar. After a period of withdrawal symptoms she began to lose weight slowly. She was then advised to avoid dairy products, soya, peanuts, hazelnuts and chemical sweeteners. This produced the desired result. She lost 25 lb. Her friends and family were amazed at the change in her weight and health.

If you work full-time or travel around a lot, these diets should prove to be easy to follow as long as you are prepared. If you make your meals the night before or in the morning, you can pack them into a container and take them with you. There is a tendency to think of sandwiches when it comes to packed lunches. However, that means missing out on all the other things that could go into a lunch box. Many of the meat dishes and nut roasts are delicious cold, and you can make up rice or millet salads with plenty of raw vegetables, nuts and seeds. A thermos of soup is also a good idea.

We are all social beings and it is important you do not curtail social engagements because of your new diet. Likewise, it may be tempting to abandon your regime to conform with everyone else. It is simply not worth it. As your health improves, you will notice your confidence increases and you will cease to waste time and energy worrying about what others may think.

Eating in restaurants is not usually too much of a trouble either. If you know what you are looking for, you can usually find sufficient for your needs. You can ask for the meat or fish without the sauce, for example, and fresh fruit for dessert. Try to resist fried food as the oil will have been overheated and usually re-used. As for a drink, there is always mineral water. Do not be afraid to ask for something different; chefs are often only too willing to oblige.

If you are travelling by plane, airlines will provide special diets without any problem if you remember to state what you want (within reason) at the time of booking your ticket.

Dinner parties could prove a little more awkward but only if you let them. You can tell your host at the time of the invitation that you are following a new diet and you are avoiding certain foods. If this is a problem, you can simply offer to take your own food.

If you have the occasional lapse with the rotation of foods you can always make adjustments and get back to your routine. It is important to go about the diet as naturally and as calmly as you can. Try not to become over obsessed or too fanatical as this will lead to a situation where the diet is controlling you rather than you being in charge of it.

The food families

For the diets in this book you need to be aware of the different food families. This is important because people often react to the 'relatives' of the food to which they are intolerant. For instance, if you are reacting to tomato you may also react to potato, green pepper, chillies and aubergine. In the case of the grass family, to which most cereals belong, we look more to the subdivisions. Many people only react to wheat or corn, the most commonly eaten cereals, for example, or to the cereals which contain gluten or gluten related substances, namely wheat, rye, barley and possibly, oats.

The food family chart

Apple apple, pear, quince, loquat, pectin, cider.

Arum dasheen, eddoes.

Aster lettuce, chicory, endive, globe and Jerusalem artichoke, dandelion, sunflower, salsify, tarragon, camomile, yarrow, safflower oil.

Banana banana, plantain, arrowroot.

Beech chestnuts.

Beef beef, veal, all cow's milk products.

Beet sugar beet, spinach, Swiss chard, beetroot, quinoa.

Birch filberts, hazelnuts, birch oil (wintergreen).

Bird all foul and game birds, including chicken, turkey, duck, goose, pigeon, quail, pheasant, partridge, grouse, eggs.

Blueberry blueberry, bilberry, cranberry.

Buckwheat buckwheat, rhubarb, sorrel, amaranth (nearest family).

Cashew cashew, pistachio, mango.

Citrus lemon, orange, grapefruit, lime, tangerine, citron.

Conifer juniper, pine nuts.

Crustacean crab, crayfish, lobster, prawn, shrimp.

Freshwater fish salmon, trout, pike, perch, bass.

Fungus mushrooms, yeast.

Ginger East Indian arrowroot, ginger, cardamom, turmeric.

Gooseberry currant, gooseberry.

Grape grapes, raisins, wine, cream of tartar.

Grass wheat, spelt wheat, corn (maize), oats, barley, rye, rice, malt, millet, bamboo shoots, sugar cane, sorghum, kamut.

Honeysuckle elderberry.

Laurel avocado, cinnamon, bay leaves.

Lily onion, garlic, asparagus, chives, leeks.

Mallow okra, hibiscus.

Melon watermelon, cantaloupe and other melons, cucumber, courgette, marrow, pumpkin, acorn squash and other squashes.

Mint apple mint, basil, bergamot, hyssop, lavender, lemon balm, marjoram, oregano, peppermint, rosemary, sage, spearmint, savory, thyme.

Mollusc abalone, snail, squid, clam, mussel, oyster, scallop, octopus.

Morning glory sweet potato.

Mulberry figs, mulberry, hops, breadfruit.

Mustard turnip, radish, horseradish, salad mustard and cress, Chinese leaves, watercress, cabbage, cauliflower, broccoli, sprouts, kohlrabi, kale, mustard seed, rape seed.

Myrtle allspice, cloves, guava.

Nutmeg nutmeg, mace.

Olive black or green olives.

Palm coconut, date, date sugar, sago.

Parsley carrots, parsnips, celery, celeriac, fennel, anise, parsley, caraway, lovage, chervil, coriander, cumin.

Pea pea, dried beans, broad beans, green beans, soybeans, lentils, liquorice, peanuts, fenugreek, red clover, senna, carob.

Pepper black and white pepper, peppercorn.

Pineapple pineapple.

Plum plum, cherry, peach, apricot, nectarine, prune, almond.

Potato potato, tomato, aubergine, peppers, paprika, cayenne, tobacco.

Rose strawberry, raspberry, blackberry, loganberry, rose-hip.

Saltwater fish tuna, mackerel, herring, eel, halibut, turbot, anchovy, sardine and pilchard, whitebait, sprats, sea bass, plaice, sole, cod, hake, haddock, sea bream, mullet.

Spurge cassava (tapioca).

Subucaya brazil nut.

Swine all pork products.

Walnut walnut, hickory nut, butternut, walnut, pecan.

Yam yam.

chapter 3 the preliminary diet

Now you have recognised many of the symptoms of your food intolerances you can move on to diagnosing them. The Elimination Diet outlined in the next chapter is based on a 28-day plan that will allow you to pin-point which foods are causing you problems. Having done this, you can then work out a diet that is right for you and so begin to build your body up to full health again. However, you may find you want to prepare yourself before embarking on the Elimination Diet. If so, the Preliminary Diet will provide a nutritious and varied diet that will give your digestive system a chance to recover. If you follow this run-in diet for three weeks you will probably find your health improves dramatically. This is because you will be eating only fresh, whole foods and, at the same time, you will also be avoiding all the common allergens.

The majority of people with allergies or food intolerances react to less than five items, of which the most common are tap water, dairy products, wheat and the other cereals that contain substances similar to gluten, namely rye, barley and oats; cane and beet sugar; corn, soya, coffee, tea, eggs, peanuts, shellfish, strawberries, tomatoes, potatoes and the other members of the potato family, onions, leeks and garlic, citrus fruits, apples, food additives and preservatives. So it is most likely that by following the Preliminary Diet you will also come off all of the foods to which you are allergic or intolerant. If you feel that this has happened, you can then skip the first week of the

Elimination Diet and go straight to Day 9 to work through the remaining foods, eliminating any to which you are allergic or intolerant and adding those to which you are not to your diet.

If, however, you are still feeling unwell, you will probably find you are reacting to some of the less likely foods. In this case, you will need to test the foods more systematically. This you can do by following the initial part of the Elimination Diet. Then, once you have worked out which foods you have been reacting to, you can continue with the plan to sort out whether there are other foods that cause you problems.

Anyone who is chronically sick or who knows they have multiple 'allergies' should start at the beginning of the 28-day plan straightaway and, if necessary, take it slower by introducing fewer foods each day.

The Preliminary Diet can include the following foods (see the basic food list on page 23 for further information about those ingredients marked with an * below):

Cereals

brown rice, brown rice flakes, flour, bran and rice pasta, millet, millet flakes, flour and pasta, tapioca and tapioca flour, quinoa and quinoa flakes, arrowroot, buckwheat, buckwheat flakes, flour and pasta, sorghum, gram flour (chickpea), lima bean flour, lentil flour, sago and sago flour, sweet potato flour, chestnut flour, green banana flour (plantain), brazil nut flour, carob.

Meats

lamb, lamb's liver and kidneys, rabbit, hare, venison, wild game.

Fish

fresh tuna, sardines and pilchards, herrings, mackerel, mullet, turbot, halibut, sprats, whitebait.

Drinks and sugars

mineral water, plain herb teas like linden, peppermint, sage, camomile, lemon balm, rose hip, fennel, Equisetum tea, African Rooibosch tea, honey, fruit sugar, rice syrup, date syrup and maple syrup.

Vegetables

choose from **the parsley food family** (carrots, parsnips, celery, celeriac, fennel); **the mustard family** (turnip, radish, daikon, Chinese leaves, watercress, mustard and cress, cabbage, cauliflower, broccoli, sprouts, kohlrabi, kale); spinach, Swiss chard; seaweed, okra; **the aster family** (lettuce, chicory, endive, globe and Jerusalem artichoke, dandelion, sunflower, salsify), **the pea family** (green beans, broad beans, peas, sugar peas, mangetout, alfalfa sprouts, chickpeas, mung beans, lentils, lima beans, black eyed beans, pinto beans, but not soya beans); **the melon family** (cucumber, pumpkin, courgette, marrow, squash), plantain, sweet potatoes, yams, eddoes, dasheen, cassava and breadfruit.

Fruit

bananas, pineapple, kiwi fruit, raspberry, blackberry, loganberry, rose-hip, blueberry, cranberry, **the plum family** (plum, cherry, peach, apricot, nectarine, prune), pears, gooseberry, red, black and white currants, melon, watermelon, cantaloupe melon, other melons, acorn, pears, figs, gooseberry, papaya, avocado pear, mango, grapes, raisins, sultanas, currants, dates.

Nuts and seeds

almonds, walnuts, pecan nuts, Brazil nuts, hazelnuts, chestnuts, tiger nuts, hickory nuts, butternuts, macedamia nuts, coconut, pine nuts, sunflower seeds, pumpkin seeds, sesame seeds and tahini.

Herbs and spices

parsley, caraway, dill, anise, fennel seeds, celery seeds, cumin, coriander, lovage, mint, basil, lemon balm, rosemary, sage, thyme, savory, marjoram, oregano, lemon verbena, lemongrass, camomile, tarragon, yarrow, borage, bay leaf, juniper berries, turmeric, ginger, nutmeg, mace, cinnamon, clove, cardamom, allspice, mustard seeds, fenugreek, liquorice.

Oils

olive oil, sunflower seed oil, safflower oil, flax seed oil (linseed), sesame seed oil, walnut oil and almond oil.

Amaranth*

Buckwheat*

Kelp*

Millet*

Quinoa*

Sorghum*

Sweet potatoes, yams, cassava, eddoes and dasheen*

Tahini*

Tapioca comes from the cassava root and is sold as pearls, flakes or as a flour and can be bought in most supermarket stores. It consists almost entirely of starch with traces of calcium and other minerals. It can be used in puddings and as a thickener in soups and sauces.

Tiger nuts tubers rather than nuts and about the size of peanuts. They are cultivated in Spain and are available at some health food stores. They can be used for making 'nut' milks and for eating raw as a snack.

Guidelines to help you through the Preliminary Diet

- Vegetables can be washed in tap water and then rinsed in mineral water. Remember to clean your teeth with mineral water and check that your toothpaste does not contain sugar or any other substance you are trying to avoid.

- It is safer to alternate fruits so that you do not eat the same fruit for more than two days in a row followed by at least two days without that particular fruit. The same applies to herbs, herb teas and tea. Use powdered ginger and other spices very sparingly and only use carob powder in the third week.

- Also take care with fruit sugar, honey, date syrup, rice syrup and maple syrup. Use very little and alternate them if necessary. Some people who are allergic to pollen may react to honey. Also try to choose honey from bees that are unlikely to have been fed on sugar throughout the winter months, such as honey from Mexico, Argentina and Australia. Cold pressed, organic honey is ideal.

- If you feel better after three weeks, you can then introduce more foods into your diet following the plan laid out in the Elimination Diet. Start at Day 9 with the introduction of tap water and then continue through until Day 28. You will find that some of the foods in those subsequent days, such as avocado pear for example, will not need to be tested as you will have already included them in the Preliminary Diet. All such foods will be marked with an asterisk so you will be able to recognise them immediately. You can simply introduce these foods into your diet as shown without having to test them.

- If, however, you do not feel any better and you have checked that you are not reacting to any chemicals or fumes, go to the beginning of the Elimination Diet procedure and start at Day 1.

The following menus are only suggestions. You can use any of the recipes in the following pages as well as those from Days 1 to 8 inclusive in the Elimination Diet.

Suggested menus for the Preliminary Diet

Monday
Breakfast
Rice flake muesli (p.84)

Main meals
Grilled mackerel or turbot with gooseberry sauce served with mashed yam and fresh salad
Quinoa nut roast (p.165) served with fresh salad

Light meals
Lentil soup (p.108) with rice bread (p.209)

Tuesday
Breakfast
Millet and buckwheat muesli (millet and buckwheat flakes, chopped almonds, sultanas, dates) with almond milk (p.235)

Main meals
Game bird casserole (p.130) served with green vegetables
Vegetable hash browns (p.90) served with fennel and bean sprout salad (p.199)

Light meals
Cream of cauliflower soup with almonds (p.92)

Wednesday
Breakfast
Millet porridge (see Quinoa porridge, p.81) with fresh banana

Main meals
Lamb burgers (p.136) served with sweet potatoes and green vegetables
Barley, cashew and vegetable loaf (p.162) served with fresh salad

Light meals
Sweet potato and seafood bakes (p.163)
Stuffed mushrooms (p.113)

Thursday
Breakfast
Quinoa porridge (p.81) with Hunza apricots

Main meals
Braised venison with juniper (p.141) served with redcurrant sauce (p.196), broccoli and sweet potatoes
Steamed vegetables (p.190) with millet (p.184)

Light meals
Celery and courgette soup (p.93)

Friday
Breakfast
Rice porridge (p.83) with fresh pears

Main meals
Red mullet with seasoned rice stuffing (p.153) served with spinach
Millet, lentil and brazil nut loaf (p.162) served with green vegetables or salad

Light meals
Green split pea soup with broccoli (p.94)

Saturday

Breakfast

Rice porridge (p.83) with fresh raspberries

Main meals

Rabbit hot pot (p.133) served with fresh green vegetables
Parsnip and walnut croquettes (p.186) served with raw salad or steamed vegetables

Light meals

Celery and chestnut soup (p.93)

Sunday

Breakfast

Fresh melon with ginger

Main meals

Wild duck with pineapple (p.128) served with sweet potatoes and cauliflower
Apricot and almond pilaff (p.166) with fresh salad

Light meals

Cream of carrot and celeriac soup (p.95)

chapter 4 the elimination diet

This diet consists of a modified fast for four days, followed by a gradual re-introduction of foods. Fasting ensures that the digestive system is rested so the body can begin to extract toxins from the cells and tissues. A pure fast would consist of taking nothing by mouth except spring water. Many people do this regularly because it makes them feel good. However, as the purpose of this diet is simply to clear your body of any possible items that may be causing adverse reactions, you do not need to eliminate all foods. Instead, you can eat foods that are very unlikely to cause any reaction and therefore toxins. Only those people familiar with fasting should attempt a water only fast as it can release toxins very quickly, often causing intense reactions.

By giving your body time to rest by fasting and cleansing, any food intolerances will start to become 'unmasked'. One of the effects of this is that any reaction to a food when re-introduced will be more acute, so foods that had little or no apparent effect on you may suddenly produce noticeable reactions. It will therefore be easy for you to work out whether a food is causing any problems. Whereas before, your body may have reacted only when run-down or under stress, and therefore less able to cope, the clearer your body becomes, the more definite the signs will be. You will also find that you can start to listen to your body and sense what it is telling you. This is an important first step to full health.

Do not be put off by the thought of having to change your daily life. Simply go about the alterations methodically and positively. Once you have bought the necessary items for your larder and store cupboard (see page 23) and eliminated the things that need to be eliminated, you can then just incorporate the changes into your routine. The difference this can make to your health and to your life can be wonderful.

Withdrawal symptoms

During the first four days of the Elimination Diet you are likely to feel unwell due to withdrawal symptoms but by Day 5 you should feel better and will be able to start the re-introduction of foods, as suggested here.

Foods are re-introduced according to their food family. When you test the foods you will be able to tell whether or not you are allergic or intolerant to them. If you react to any foods you should then avoid them. The recipes have been designed to make this as easy as possible for you. If you do not react, you can then simply introduce them into your diet as the plan shows you. You may notice that some foods will not be introduced into the diet immediately after testing. This is simply a precaution in case you react more slowly to them as people sometimes do. The majority of foods, though, will produce immediately recognisable symptoms.

Symptoms might well vary from food to food. Some foods will produce more severe reactions and others, more delayed and the types of symptoms can also differ enormously. Sometimes, for example, you may experience panic attacks, other times just a faint headache. This is where the pulse test is invaluable (see page 18). Do not forget to use this and then to record all reactions in your food diary (see page 16).

Guidelines to help you through the Elimination Diet

- If you can, try to test the foods in as many different ways as possible – raw, lightly cooked and cooked slowly for a longer time as this may make a difference as to whether or not you react. The recipes and the menus have been designed to help you to do this. Do not worry, though, if you cannot test all the members of each food family (see page 31). There are, of course, exceptions to the rule, but normally if you react to one member of a family, you will do so to all the others. Those that are the normal exceptions have been introduced separately into the 28-Day plan.

- For those with multiple food intolerances, it may be that you will need to slow down the diet a little. For some people, just introducing one new food or food family at a time, will be sufficient. Remember that this is a diet about getting well, not about racing to the end. If you are unsure about a reaction you can leave the food family out and test again in four day's time.

- You may find that you are trying out new foods that you have not eaten before. This is a good idea, not only because it offers you delicious new foods but will also mean your diet may not be as limited as it might if you have to start avoiding certain foods. So try the quails eggs, the venison

---

Case study

Sandra was always in trouble at school. She fell asleep over her desk, never did her homework and frequently arrived late. Her school demanded that Sandra see a psychologist who suggested that she was taking 'social' drugs. Her parents knew this was wrong, however, and decided to check for allergies instead. Sandra was found to be reacting to milk produce, corn, potato, tomato, tea and particularly car fumes. Steps were taken to deal with all this and Sandra never fell asleep at school again.

and the tiger nuts, for example. They are delicious and a way of ensuring you do not feel you are depriving yourself.

■ Once you have completed the Elimination Diet you will have discovered which foods you are reacting to and you can avoid these items so your system can have a rest. In this way it will have a chance to recover and re-balance. You may want to make a list of all the foods you have had a reaction to and note the severity of the reaction. If the reaction was only a minor one, you may find you can eat it on an occasional basis, perhaps once a week, or in the following Rotation Diet. Foods that cause major reactions, though, will need to be avoided for two to three months before being tested again.

The 28-day Elimination Diet plan

DAY 1
Rice
Pears
Lamb or lentils

DAY 2
Rice
Pears
Lamb or lentils

DAY 3
Rice
Pears
Lamb or lentils
Equisetum tea

DAY 4
Rice
Pears
Lamb or lentils
Linden leaf tea

DAY 5
Rice
Lamb
Mustard family
Kiwi fruit
Flax seed oil
    (linseed)

DAY 6
Quinoa
Fish: Oily saltwater
Sweet potato
Arum family
Mallow family
Melon family
Gooseberry family
Olive oil
Mint family tea
Fruit sugar

DAY 7
Buckwheat family
Millet, tapioca
Game bird
Walnut family
Tiger nuts
Parsley family
Banana family
Pineapple, papaya
Walnut oil
Fennel tea
Maple syrup

DAY 8
Sago
Sorghum
Yam
Rabbit, hare
Aster family
Plum family
Sunflower oil
Safflower oil
Almond oil
Honey
Camomile tea

DAY 9
Rice
Lamb
Tap water
Pea family (not
    soya)
Pears, quince,
    loquat Lychees
Brazil nuts
Macadamia nuts
Lemon verbena tea
Fenugreek tea

DAY 10
Barley
Fish: Saltwater
Venison
Beet family, olives
Rose family
Conifer family
Pumpkin seeds
Mulberry family
Cashew family
Lemongrass tea
Raspberry leave tea

DAY 11
Quail, Quail's eggs
Lily family
Laurel family
Citrus family
Blueberry family
Chestnuts
Birch family
Taheebo Tea (Pau
    Darco)
Orange juice
Rice syrup

DAY 12
Beef and veal
Potato family
Grape family
Seaweed
Palm family
Sesame seeds and
    oil
Date syrup

DAY 13
Pork, wild boar
Soya products
Mushrooms
Apples, pectin
Mustard seed

DAY 14
Oats
Fish: Freshwater
Ginger family
Nutmeg family

DAY 15
Turkey
Rooibosch tea
Myrtle family
Black and white
  pepper

DAY 16
Corn
Chicory coffee
Dandelion coffee
Barleycup

DAY 17
Yeast
Green leaf tea

DAY 18
Rye
Fish: Crustacean
  family

DAY 19
Duck, goose
Duck's eggs, goose
  eggs

DAY 20
Sheep's milk
  products

DAY 21
Cane sugar
Wine vinegar

DAY 22
Wheat, Spelt wheat
Kamut
Fish: Mollusc
  family

DAY 23
Chicken
Chicken's eggs

DAY 24
Goat's milk
  products

DAY 25
Tea
Peanuts
Cider vinegar

DAY 26
Cocoa

DAY 27
Coffee

DAY 28
Cow's milk
  products

Days 1 to 4

Eat any of the following:

Pears

Rice

Lamb or lentils

Sea salt

Mineral water

Equisetum (horsetail) and **linden leaf tea** on Days 3 and 4.

▦ If you suffer from arthritis, you may find that red meat is too acidic for you. In which case you may want to avoid lamb altogether and substitute lentils or maybe the mustard family.

▦ **It is very important to exclude everything else from your diet.** A small drink of tea or coffee could alter the whole experiment and you would need to start again. This also includes smoking. This may seem extreme, but it is worth persevering. The diet is for a relatively short amount of time and it can bring a lifetime's benefit.

Suggested menu

On rising

Drink 2 glasses of hot water

8am   1 to 2 fresh pears

10am   Grilled lamb or a serving of lentils and rice

1pm   Lamb with rice or lentils with rice

4pm   Fresh pear

6pm   Rice porridge with cooked pears

9pm   Fresh pear

Day 5

Introduce and test the following:

The mustard family: turnip, swede, radish, daikon, watercress, mustard and cress, Chinese leaves, cabbage, cauliflower, broccoli, sprouts, kohlrabi, kale.

Kiwi fruit

Flax seed oil (linseed oil): This may be sprinkled on salads or added to mashed vegetable but do not use this oil for cooking. Lamb dripping can be saved for this purpose.

Suggested menu

Breakfast

Fresh pears with rice porridge (p.83)

Vegetable hash browns (p.90)

Main meal

Grilled lamb with green vegetables and mashed swede

Rice and lentils with green vegetables and mashed swede

Light meal

Turnip and watercress soup (p.94)

Steamed vegetables with rice

Raw salad

Sliced Chinese leaves, watercress, mustard and cress, radishes or grated daikon dressed with safflower oil

Fruit

Pears

Kiwi fruit

Drinks

Mineral water

Linden leaf tea

Rice milk (p.234)

Day 6

You now need to come off rice, pears, lentils and lamb in order to test them on Day 9.

Soak tiger nuts overnight for Day 7.

Introduce and test the following:

Quinoa

Sweet potato, dasheen and eddoe

Fruit sugar

Olive oil

Saltwater fish: mackerel, sardine, herring, fresh tuna, anchovy, halibut, turbot, red or grey mullet, whitebait.

The mallow family: Okra, hibiscus.

The melon family: watermelon, cantaloupe and other melons, cucumber, courgette, marrow, pumpkin, acorn squash and other squashes.

The gooseberry family: gooseberry, red-, white- and blackcurrants.

The mint family: fresh peppermint tea, sage, basil, lemon balm, thyme, rosemary, marjoram, oregano.

Suggested menu

Breakfast

Melon

Quinoa porridge (p.81) with stewed gooseberries or kiwi fruit

Main meal

Grilled sardines with baked sweet potato and cucumber salad

Grilled mackerel, with gooseberry sauce and cucumber salad

Light meal

Sweet potato and seafood bakes (p.163)

Raw salad

Cucumbers and suitable vegetables from the mustard family and okra

Fruit

Melon

Stewed or raw blackcurrants or gooseberries

Drinks

Mineral water

Peppermint, lemon balm, sage, thyme, rosemary and hibiscus tea.

Day 7

Prepare and soak the lentils and beans today that you wish to use
on Day 9.

Introduce and test the following:

Millet

Cassava (tapioca)

Maple syrup

The buckwheat family: buckwheat, rhubarb, sorrel, amaranth.

Wild game bird: pigeon, wild duck, partridge, grouse, pheasant.

Walnuts, pecan nuts, hickory nut, butternut, tiger nuts
Walnut oil

The parsley family: carrots, parsnips, celery, celeriac, fennel,
anise, parsley, caraway, dill, cumin, coriander, lovage.

The banana family: banana, plantain, arrowroot.

Pineapple

Papaya

NB: Nuts and seeds can be tested on their own, before adding to recipes.

Suggested menu

Breakfast

Diced pineapple and banana fruit salad

Millet porridge (p.81) or Buckwheat muesli (p.85) with pecan nuts,
banana and tiger nut milk (p.233)

(Millet and millet porridge can be cooked in the same way as quinoa
or you can use millet flakes. Buckwheat and millet flakes may be
used to make up the muesli.)

Main meal

Game bird casserole (p.130) with broccoli, sprouts or other green vegetables

Parsnip and walnut croquettes (p.186) served with carrots and green vegetables

Light meals

Cream of carrot and celeriac soup (p.95)

Celery, walnut and fennel salad with buckwheat pasta

Grated carrot, celery and nut salad with millet

Puddings

Baked bananas with chopped pecan nuts and maple syrup

Drinks

Mineral water

Fennel tea

Day 8

Test and introduce the following foods into your diet:

Yam, sago, sorghum

Rabbit, hare

The Aster family: lettuce, chicory, endive, salsify, globe and Jerusalem artichoke, dandelion, sunflower seeds, tarragon, camomile, yarrow.

The Plum family: plum, cherry, peach, apricot, nectarine, prune, almond.

Sunflower, safflower oil and almond oil

Camomile tea

Honey

Suggested menu
Breakfast
Fresh peaches and cherries
Quinoa or sorghum porridge (p.81 and 82) with cooked Hunza or
un-sulphured apricots and almonds

Main meal
Turkey and apricot pilaff (p.127) with lettuce salad

Light meal
Yam and chicory soup (p.95)
Boiled yam with lettuce and chicory salad

Day 9

Test **rice** and re-introduce on Day 11 if no adverse reactions have
been experienced.

Introduce and test the following:
*Pears, quince, loquat and lychees
*Lamb
*The pea family: peas, sugar peas, mangetout, green beans,
broad beans, dried beans (chickpeas, black eyed beans, pinto
beans, mung beans, aduki beans, lentils, alfalfa sprouts, mung
bean sprouts – but test soya on Day 13 and peanuts on Day 25).
*Brazil nuts
*Macedamia nuts
*Lemon verbena tea
*Fenugreek tea
Tap water: test this at the end of the day and if this is all right
you may start using filtered tap water instead of mineral water.

Suggested menu
Breakfast
Pears
Millet and buckwheat flakes (p.85) with lychees or kiwi fruit

Main meals

Grilled lamb with peas or green beans and sweet potato

Light meals

Lentil soup (p.108) with rice cakes

Brazil nut bean burgers (p.164) with green salad

Boiled rice for testing (p.184)

Day 10

Test **barley** at the end of the day and introduce on Day 12 if no adverse reaction has been experienced.

Introduce and test the following:

*Venison

Saltwater fish: cod, haddock, hake, plaice, sole, sea bream, whiting.

*The beet family: spinach, Swiss chard, beetroot, beet sugar (test only).

The rose family: strawberry, *raspberry, *blackberry, *loganberry, *rose-hip.

*The conifer family: pine nuts, juniper berries.

*Cashew family: cashew nuts, pistachio nuts, mango.

*Mulberry: figs, hops, mulberries, breadfruit

*Pumpkin seeds

*Olives

*Lemongrass tea

*Raspberry leaf tea

Suggested menu

Breakfast

Compote of fresh strawberries and raspberries mixed with cooked blackberries

Quinoa porridge (p.81)

Main meal

Braised venison with juniper (page 141) served with redcurrant sauce, sautéed sweet potatoes and spinach

Rolled plaice with spinach (p.154) served with carrots

Butternut squash with pine nuts (p.186) served with sweet potatoes

Light meals

Swiss chard and celery soup (p.96) with barley scone bread (p.208)

Millet and cashew nut risotto (p.161) served with melon, strawberry and cucumber salad (p.200)

Day 11

If you have had no adverse reaction to testing rice on Day 9 you can now start using it again in your diet.

Introduce and test the following:

Quail

Quail's eggs

The lily family: onion, garlic, asparagus, chives, leeks.

The citrus family: lemon, orange, grapefruit, lime, tangerine, citron.

*The blueberry family: blueberry, cranberry.

*The laurel family: avocado, cinnamon, bay leaves.

*The beech family: chestnuts and chestnut flour.

*The birch family: filberts, hazelnuts.

*Taheebo (Pau Darco) tea

Orange juice

*Rice syrup

Suggested menu

Breakfast

Fresh grapefruit

Millet and kamut porridge (p.82)

Poached quail's eggs with sweet potato or yam

Main meal

Roast quails with spring onion rice and cranberry sauce (p.131) and served with green vegetables

Brussels sprouts with chestnuts (p.187) served with millet

Egg and pasta salad (p.200) with a French dressing (p.197)

Light meals

Cream of asparagus soup (p.97)

Avocado pear with French dressing (p.197)

Day 12

Introduce **barley.**

Test and introduce the following:

Beef, veal

The potato family: potato, tomato, aubergine, peppers, paprika, cayenne.

*The palm family: coconut, date, date syrup.

*Grapes, raisins, sultanas

*Seaweed

*Sesame seeds and spread (tahini)

*Sesame seed oil

Suggested menu

Breakfast

Grapes

Rice porridge with prunes (p.83)

Barley/rice and sesame seed snacks (p.87)

Main meals

Beef stew and barley dumplings (p.144) served with mashed potatoes and peas

Vegetable goulash (p.167) with barley dumplings (p.193)

Light meals

Baked tomato soup (p.98) with barley scone bread (p.208)

Green pepper and pine nut pizza (p.168) with salad

Day 13

Introduce and test the following:

Soya and soya bean products: soya flour, soya milk, soya dried milk, soya oil, soya meat substitutes, tofu, tempeh, soya egg replacer, tamari soya sauce.

Wild boar and outdoor reared pork

Apples and pectin: some sugar-free jams are made with apple juice and pectin.

Mushrooms: including wild porcini, oyster and shiitake.

*Mustard seed

Suggested menu

Breakfast

Fresh apples

Rice porridge (p.83) with stewed apples and raisins and soya milk (p.236)

Main meal

Wild boar cutlets with mushroom sauce (p.151) served with French beans and yam

Pork, apple and chestnut pie (soya mince may be substituted for pork) (p.146), served with seasonal vegetables or salad

Light meal

Yellow split pea soup (p.99)

Smoked tofu and mushroom kebabs (p.167) with fresh salad

Day 14

Test **oats** and introduce on Day 16.

Introduce the following:
Freshwater fish: salmon, trout, pike, perch, bass.
*Ginger family: arrowroot, acrimony, cardamom, ginger, turmeric.
*Nutmeg family: nutmeg, mace.

Suggested menu
Breakfast
Fresh melon with ground ginger and fruit sugar
Pear and ginger fruit slice (p.89)

Main meals
Fresh salmon with raspberry coulis (p.156) served with rice and French beans
Cardamom nut rice (p.185) with fresh green salad

Light meals
Stuffed papayas (p.187)
Breadfruit with ginger and green peppers (p.169)

Day 15

Introduce and test the following:
Turkey
*The myrtle family: allspice, cloves, guava.
Black and white pepper: this can be used uncooked, on cold food. When it is cooked, however, pepper can become an irritant and is not good for the liver.
*Rooibosch tea: this is an African tea available at health food stores and some supermarkets. It is additive and caffeine free and low in tannin and may be made like ordinary tea and served with a slice of lemon.

You can have quail's eggs again today but do not use them again until you have tested duck's eggs on Day 19. This is to give you a four-day gap.

Suggested menu
Breakfast
Freshly squeezed orange juice
Buckwheat muesli (p.85) with millet
Poached or scrambled quail's eggs

Main meals
Turkey and mushroom fricassée (p.126) with sautéed sweet potato and fresh green salad (p.198)
Cauliflower and chick pea curry (p.175) with wholemeal basmati rice and sliced tomatoes

Light meals
Onion and barley soup (p.96)
Stuffed baked potato (p.180) with coleslaw (p.201)

Day 16
Test **corn** (cornflour, maize flour, sweetcorn), and introduce on Day 18.
You can introduce oats, providing you have not had any adverse reactions.
If you wish, you can introduce barleycup, chicory and dandelion coffee substitutes. Chicory and dandelion belong to the Aster family.

Suggested menu
Breakfast
Fresh fruit
Oat milk (p.233)
Old-fashioned oatmeal porridge (p.82)
Date and coconut muesli bars (p.218)

Main meals
Shoulder of lamb with raisin, apricot and oat stuffing (p.138) with new potatoes and seasonal green vegetables
Green pepper and aubergine flan (p.171) served with arame seaweed with sesame seeds (p.199) and fresh green salad (p.198)

Light meals
Miso soup (p.98) with corn bread (p.208)
Hummus and cannellini bean dip (p.118) with crudités

Day 17

Test and introduce **yeast** and **green leaf tea,** which is a china tea, low in caffeine and tannin. It is drunk without milk but may be served with lemon.

Suggested menu
Breakfast
Pears and rice porridge (p.83)
Barley muffins (p.218)

Main meal
Venison steak burgers (p.141) with mixed vegetables and salad

Light meals
Mushroom and black bean soup (p.100)
Rice, barley and bean sprout salad (p.201)

Day 18

Introduce **corn,** providing you have not had any adverse reactions.
Test **rye** and introduce on Day 20.
NB: If you buy rye/pumpernickel bread, check that it does not contain any wheat.

Introduce and test the following:
The crustacean family: crab, crayfish, lobster, prawn, shrimp.

Suggested menu

Breakfast

Fresh melon

Quinoa porridge (p.81) with ginger syrup (p.195)

Main meals

Prawn, avocado and fennel salad with buckwheat pasta (p.202)

Stuffed green peppers (p.191) served with baby corn and sugar peas

Light meals

Sweetcorn and lima bean succotash soup (p.107) with rye crackers

Open sandwiches using pumpernickel rye bread (p.122)

Day 19

Test **duck and goose** and **duck's eggs and goose eggs,** but do not introduce duck's eggs into your diet until you have tested chicken's eggs on Day 23. You can continue to have duck after today, though, provided you have had no adverse reactions.

Suggested menu

Breakfast

Orange and grapefruit salad

Buckwheat muesli (p.85) with millet

Main meals

Roast duck with orange and grapefruit sauce (p.129) with runner beans or seasonal vegetables

Millet, hazelnut and tofu croquettes (p.193) with tomato sauce (p.196) served with vegetables

Light meals

Celery and chestnut soup (see page 93)

Stuffed tomatoes (see page 114)

Day 20

Test **sheep's milk products** but do not introduce into your diet until after Day 28 when you will have tested cow's milk yoghurt and cheese.

Rye can now be introduced providing you are clear of any adverse reaction.

Suggested menu

Breakfast

Fresh fruit with sheep's milk yoghurt

Rye crackers with sheep's cheese and alfalfa sprouts

Main meals

Creamy lamb with rye spaghetti (p.139)

Fresh green salad

Baked beans in tomato sauce (p.179) served with baked potatoes and fresh green salad

Light meals

Leek and potato soup (p.100) with rye bread (p.211)

Greek salad (p.203)

Day 21

Test **cane sugar,** but do not introduce.

Introduce and test **wine vinegar.**

Suggested menu

Breakfast

Fresh fruit

Compote of mixed dried fruit (figs, prunes, pears, apricots) with oat flakes

Main meals

Pork tenderloin with prune, anchovy and almond stuffing (p.147) served with rice, carrots and peas

Sweet and sour vegetables/pork (p.148) served with basmati wholemeal rice

Light meals

Green split pea soup with broccoli (p.94)

Stuffed mushrooms (p.113)

Day 22

Test **wheat** (spelt wheat and kamut if available) and introduce in 2 days time on Day 24 providing you have had no adverse reactions. **Spelt wheat** is an ancient precursor of modern day wheat and is often more easily tolerated. **Kamut** is an ancient, non-hybridised grain, now being produced in the United States and slowly coming on to the market in Great Britain. It is a variety of high-protein, low gluten wheat. It is usually tolerated well by 'wheat allergic' people.

Introduce and test following:

The mollusc family: abalone, snail, squid, clam, mussel, oyster, scallop, octopus.

Suggested menu

Breakfast

Fresh fruit

Lamb burgers (p.136)

Main meals

Seafood paella (p.160) with fresh green salad

Vegetable and lentil dal (p.174) with bulgur wheat (p.191) (for testing) or millet

Light meals

Spiced pumpkin and ginger soup (p.104) with organic wholemeal bread (for testing)

Tortillas with sweetcorn and tomato filling (p.116) served with fresh green salad

Day 23

Introduce and test **chicken** and **chicken's eggs**. Providing you have not experienced any adverse reactions, you can now use all eggs including quail's and duck's in your diet.

Suggested menu

Breakfast

Fresh fruit

Tropical fruit muesli

Boiled egg

Main meal

Curried chicken (p.125) with rice, buckwheat chappatis (p.212) and sliced tomatoes or pineapple chunks

Sweet potato and parsnip bakes (p.176) served with fresh green salad

Light meal

Garden vegetable soup (p.101)

Avocado sweet and sour salad (p.204)

Day 24

Introduce and test **goat's milk products:** goat's milk, cheese and live yoghurt.

Suggested menu

Breakfast

Fresh fruit with goat's milk yoghurt

Scrambled egg on toast

Main meals

Chilli con carne (p.145) served with long grain rice and fresh green salad (p.198)

Lamb or vegetable moussaka (p.140) with fresh green salad (p.198)

Light meals

Cream of artichoke soup (p.101)

Day 25

Test **tea** and **cider vinegar**. You can also test **peanuts,** but take care not to eat too many because they may contain carcinogenic substances made by a fungus to which they are very susceptible.

Suggested menu

Breakfast

Fresh apple, pear or lychees

Corn flakes (organic) with soya or nut milk (pages 230-236)

Main meals

Fruit-roasted leg of wild boar (p.152) with mashed potato, baked red cabbage (p.190) and garden peas

Root vegetable crumble (p.177) with baked red cabbage (p.177) and green vegetables

Light meals

Celery and courgette soup (p.93)

Barley, cashew and vegetable loaf (p.162) with fennel and bean sprout salad (p.199)

Tofu mayonnaise (p.195)

Day 26

Test **cocoa**. Chocolate bars made from organically grown cocoa beans can be bought at most health food stores.

Suggested menu
Breakfast
Fresh fruit
Chocolate hazelnut biscuits (p.222)

Main meals
Pot roast leg of lamb (p.137) served with mashed potato and broccoli
Kedgeree (p.178) served with fresh spinach and carrots
Millet, lentil and brazil nut loaf (p.162)

Light meals
Salmon and tomato fish cakes (p.156)
Prawn or tofu chow mein (p.157)

Day 27

Test **coffee**. Use filtered organic coffee (instant coffee contains chemicals). Coffee is a stimulant and can increase any adverse response that may be occurring, so only drink in moderation, if at all.

Suggested menu
Breakfast
Avocado fruit cocktail (p.89)
Sprouted grain bread (p.212)

Main meals
Chicken noodle main meal soup (p.102)
Wild duck with pineapple (p.128) served with braised celery (p.192)
Spanish omelette (p.161) served with boiled potatoes and fresh green salad

Light meals
Broccoli with ginger and macadamia nuts (p.188) served with couscous (or quinoa)

Day 28

Test and introduce the following:

Cow's milk and **cow's milk products**: yoghurt, cheese, cream, butter and ghee (clarified butter). Clarified butter can often be tolerated by milk-sensitive people. This is because the milk protein, traces of which are found in butter, have been separated. It can be bought as Ghee at Indian food shops and at most supermarkets. It can also be made at home by melting a pack of butter over gentle heat, allowing it to cook slightly and then pouring off the liquid into a glass jar. The proteins in the butter will then have settled on the bottom of the pan.

Suggested menu

Breakfast
Fresh fruit with organic cow's milk yoghurt
Celebration carrot cake (p.214)

Main meals
Lamb noisettes (p.135) with a cheesy rice topping, garnished with mushrooms and served with seasonal green vegetables
Vegetarian/lamb shepherd's pie (p.136) served with green vegetables

Light meals
Minestrone soup (p.103)
Stuffed baked potatoes (p.180) with choice of fillings and fresh green salad (p.198)

chapter 5 the rotation diet

Having established which foods you are reacting to, it is now helpful to follow a Rotation Diet. The purpose of a Rotation Diet is to prevent the development of new allergies and intolerances to foods. Often people find that if they avoid the foods to which they are allergic or intolerant, they experience a great improvement in their health initially but can then start to feel unwell again. This is because they have become allergic or intolerant to something else in the meantime – often a substitute food, which they have eaten too frequently. For example, it is common for someone to replace cow's milk with soya milk, only to find they then develop an intolerance to soya. In addition, a Rotation Diet can also reduce existing food allergies and intolerances as it allows the body to process each food properly. Hence it is a way for many people to overcome their intolerances and, for those with multiple food allergies and intolerances, it can often mean they can include more items in their diet than they may otherwise be able to do.

On average, it takes three days for a meal to pass through the human digestive system and to be processed by the body, so to be safe the diet is based on a four-day plan. For example, if you were to eat wheat on Monday, you would then not have it again until Thursday.

With the exception of the Grass family, when foods are rotated, it is the whole food family to which the particular food belongs that is rotated (see page 31). This is important because people can cross-react to the 'relatives' of a food to which they are intolerant. For instance, if you are intolerant to onion, you may suspect leek, garlic, chives and possibly asparagus. For more information see pages 31-33.

You will need to avoid foods that you know cause reactions. The recipes have been designed to make it easy for you to leave out any of the foods you cannot tolerate and perhaps substitute other foods that you can. You may also find that as your body clears, small sensitivities that had previously been masked, may appear. In this case, you will need to avoid these as well.

However, if you have multiple allergies or intolerances and therefore have a very limited diet, you may have to eat some of the foods that cause the least reactions. If so, it is best to limit these to just once in the particular day. Alternatively, you may find you can tolerate some foods if eaten less frequently; once in eight days, for example.

As the weeks go by and you feel your health improving, you could try to introduce a suspect food into your diet plan. It may very well be that as your body clears, so do your allergies and food intolerances. It is likely then that foods to which you previously reacted may no longer cause you any problems. If this is so, you can simply incorporate the food into your Rotation Diet. As long as you continue to rotate those foods, you should find they remain safe foods for you.

This diet, therefore, may seem slightly tricky at first but the benefits are numerous and long-lasting. It is possible to recover your health from an allergy or food intolerance problem and a Rotation Diet should prove to be an important part of such a recovery.

Making changes in your diet

Once you have mastered the principles, you may want to rearrange some of the food families. If, for example, you wanted to make a chicken and mushroom pie, you could move the mushrooms from Day 1 to Day 3. You would do this simply by avoiding mushrooms on Day 1 and then having them on Day 3. You then need to wait at least three more days before you could eat them again. If you wanted to move them back to Day 1, you would need to avoid them on the following Day 1 and then re-introduce them on the subsequent Day 1. If you then wanted to switch avocado from Day 2 to Day 4 you would need to remember that cinnamon and bay leaves belong to the same family as avocado. So you would have to wait until the Day 4 before you could eat any of them.

Case study

Jim had suffered from fatigue which at times turned into complete exhaustion, since the age of nine. He had been an athlete in his school team but when he became unable to walk very far, he had to leave the team. He then found he could not concentrate and was unable to do his school work. He felt continually ill as if he had a viral illness. The doctor thought he was depressed and at one point recommended he should leave home and attend a psychiatric centre. His parents did not agree with this diagnosis and kept Jim at home. His parents then heard about the work of clinical ecologists in America and they visited a clinic in New York. The advice given was to follow an elimination diet. A lot of vitamin and mineral supplements were also recommended as well as amino acids, enzymes and glandular substances. The family started on the diet and on Day 5, Jim felt much better. He gradually became stronger and began to be able to concentrate. Over the next few months there were several relapses. The family discovered a clinic using clinical ecological methods in England. Each time he relapsed, more foods were found to be causing symptoms. The family were then taught how to plan a rotation diet so that no food was eaten too frequently. This solved a lot of the problems and Jim was able to study again. In 1989 Jim finished a university degree. During his four years of study he cooked his own food and kept to a rotation diet. He attended social functions taking his food with him, and then went on to full-time work. Jim realises that without a knowledge of rotation diets he might still be getting the wrong diagnoses and treatment, and he doubts if he would ever have completed his education.

The 4-day Rotation Diet plan

Day	1	2	3	4
Cereals and grains	Millet Wheat, spelt wheat Barley Rye Kamut	Corn (maize) Oats Sorghum Arrowroot	Rice Wild rice Quinoa Sago flour Any pulse flour	Amaranth Buckwheat Tapioca Chestnut flour
Meat	Rabbit/Hare Crustacean family Mollusc family Freshwater fish Yeast	Pork, Wild boar Venison	Bird family Eggs	Beef, Veal Lamb Saltwater fish Dairy products
Nuts and seeds	Cashew family Sesame	Brazil nuts Pine nuts Macadamia nuts Tiger nuts Pumpkin seeds Hemp seeds	Almond Coconut Sunflower	Hazelnut Chestnut Walnut family Poppy seeds
Sugars	Malt barley Cane sugar	Fruit sugar Corn syrup Oat syrup	Honey Date syrup Beet sugar Rice syrup	Maple syrup Apple/pear concentrate
Drinks	Tea Green leaf tea	Oat milk Hibiscus tea Mint teas Lemon verbena	Soya milk Rice milk Rooibosch tea Cocoa	Sheep's milk Goat's milk Coffee Equisetum tea
Vegetables	Parsley family Seaweed, kelp Mushrooms	Mallow family Melon family Potato family Lily family Laurel family Olives	Aster family Beet family Pea family	Arum family Mustard family Sweet potato Yam Sorrel
Herbs and spices	Parsley family Pepper family	Mint family Ginger family Juniper berries	Tarragon Fenugreek Nutmeg family	Lemongrass Myrtle family Capers
Fruit	Citrus family Blueberry family Mulberry family Elderberry Pomegranate Passion fruit Papaya Mango	Gooseberry family Banana family Pineapple	Kiwi fruit Plum family Dates Cape gooseberries Grape family	Apple family Rose family Guava Lychees Rhubarb
Oils etc. (should be cold pressed and glass bottled)	Sesame oil Wheatgerm oil	Olive oil Hemp seed oil Flax seed (linseed) oil	Sunflower oil Safflower oil Soya oil Almond oil Tropical oils Wine vinegar Balsamic	vinegar Walnut oil Hazelnut oil Cider vinegar Raspberry vinegar

Day 1

The following foods can be eaten:

Cereals: wheat, semolina and couscous (wheat), bulgur wheat, spelt wheat flour, kamut, barley, rye, ryevita, pumpernickel bread, millet; wheat, rye, barley, millet and kamut pasta.

Meat, fish etc.: rabbit and hare; the crustacean family (crab, crayfish, lobster, prawn, shrimp); the mollusc family (abalone, snail, squid, clam, mussel, oyster, octopus, scallop); freshwater fish (salmon, trout, pike, perch, bass); barley miso; yeast.

Nuts & seeds: cashew nuts, pistachio nuts; sesame seeds and spread (tahini).

Sugars: barley malt, cane sugar.

Drinks: barley cup, tea, green leaf tea, Maté tea, fennel tea, lime tea, orange juice.

Vegetables: the parsley family (carrots, parsnips, celery, celeriac, fennel); seaweed, kelp; mushrooms.

Herbs and spices: aniseed, caraway, dill, cumin, coriander, chervil, fennel leaf or seed.

Fruit: the citrus family (lemon, orange, grapefruit, lime, tangerine, citron); mango, papaya, star fruit, passion fruit, pomegranate; fig, breadfruit, mulberry; cranberry, blueberry; elderberry.

Oils: sesame seed oil, wheat germ oil.

Suggested menus

Breakfasts

Grapefruit and orange fruit salad

Frumenty (p.86)

Millet and kamut porridge (p.82)

Barley flake muesli (p.84)

Grilled trout fillets with tropical fruit (p.90)

Soups and starters

Mushroom and barley broth (p.105)

Parsnip and coriander soup (p.105)

Clear vegetable and nori broth (p.106)

the allergy exclusion diet

Fish and fennel soup (p.106)
Pistachio and rabbit/liver pâté (p.111)
Stuffed mushrooms (p.113)

Main meal dishes
Pot roast rabbit with mushroom and fennel stuffing (p.134)
Rabbit/hare hot pot (p.133)
Grilled trout fillets with tropical fruit (p.158)
Stuffed squid (p.159)

Vegetarian main meals
Millet croquettes (p.179)
Barley, cashew and vegetable loaf (p.162)
Cashew nut and celery flan (p.170)
Mixed vegetable terrine (p.181)

Vegetables and salads
Salad dressing (p.198)
Orange and fennel salad (p.203)
Braised celery (p.192)
Mixed grain salad (p.205)
Seafood salad (p.206)

Puddings and desserts
Fig and lime sorbet (p.224)
Blood oranges with cranberries (p.224)
Pistachio nut semolina with lime (p.225)

Breads, cakes and biscuits
Soda bread (p.210), Pitta bread (p.213)
Sprouted grain bread (p.212)
Barley and cashew nut scones (p.219)
Rye bread (p.211)
Carrot and fig slice (p.221)
Orange and cashew nut crunchies (p.222)

Drinks and miscellaneous

Cashew nut milk (p.234)

Carrot and cashew nut spread (p.237)

Mushroom and tahini spread (p.237)

Lemon and orange barley water (p.230)

Lemon and elderflower cordial (p.2321)

Elderberry punch (p.231)

Day 2

The following foods can be eaten:

Cereals: maize flour, cornflour, corn pasta, sorghum, arrowroot, oats, oatmeal, oat cakes, green banana flour.

Meats etc.: pork, wild boar, venison.

Nuts & seeds: Brazil nuts and spread, tiger nuts, macadamia nuts, pine nuts, pumpkin seeds, hemp seeds.

Sugars: fruit sugar, corn syrup, oat syrup.

Drinks: peppermint tea, mint tea, thyme tea, sage tea, lemon verbena and lemon balm tea, blackcurrant leaf tea, hibiscus tea.

Vegetables: avocado pear, cucumber, marrow, pumpkin, courgette, okra, plantain potato, tomato, aubergine, peppers, onion, leek, garlic, sweetcorn.

Herbs and spices: cayenne pepper, paprika pepper, ginger, turmeric, cardamom, cinnamon, bay, mint, basil, sage, oregano, thyme, rosemary, lemon balm, chives.

Fruit: banana, melon, kiwi, currants, gooseberry, pineapple.

Oils: virgin olive oil, flax seed oil, hemp seed oil.

Suggested menus

Breakfast

Melon salad

Oat flake muesli (p.85)

Old fashioned oatmeal porridge (p.82)

Speedy oat porridge (p.81)

Sorghum porridge (p.82)

Polenta (p.86)

Soups and starters
Baked tomato soup (p.98)
Avocado and green pepper soup (p.104)
Spiced pumpkin and ginger soup (p.104)
Gazpacho (p.109)
Tortillas with sweetcorn and tomato filling (p.116)
Avocado and courgette dip (p.117)

Main meals
Pork and pineapple kebabs (p.149)
Roast pork/wild boar with juniper (p.151)
Pig's liver and onions (p.149)
Venison and cucumber stir-fry (p.142)
Meatballs in tomato sauce (p.150)

Vegetarian main meals
Polenta with tomato and pepper sauce (p.182)
Green pepper and aubergine flan (p.171)
Brazil nut roast (p.164)

Vegetables and salads
Cucumber, avocado and asparagus salad (p.204)
Greek style onions (p.189)
Baked plantains (p.193)
Baked vegetables (p.189)

Puddings and desserts
Pineapple upside-down cake (p.214)
Grilled pineapple with macadamia nuts (p.226)
Fruit crêpes (p.226)

Cakes and biscuits
Green banana and oatmeal scones (p.220)
Brazil nut cookies (p.223)

Drinks and miscellaneous
Tiger nut milk (p.233)
Oat milk (p.233)
Hemp seed milk (p.233)
Banana milk shake (p.232)
Brazil nut butter (p.237)
Hemp seed butter (p.238)

Day 3

The following foods can be eaten:

Cereals: brown rice, brown rice flakes, flour and bran, rice pasta, rice cakes, rice biscuits, wild rice, quinoa, quinoa flakes and flour, sago, sago flour, soya flour, lentil flour, gram flour (chick pea), any other pulse flour.

Meat etc.: chicken and eggs, duck and eggs, quail and eggs, turkey, pigeon and any other game bird, tofu, tempeh, rice or soya miso, Umeboshi plum dressing, Tamari soya sauce.

Nuts & seeds: coconut, almonds, sunflower seeds (not peanuts).

Sugars: honey, rice syrup, date syrup, beet sugar.

Drinks: chicory coffee, dandelion root chip coffee, Rooibosch African tea, soya milk, cocoa, carob, camomile tea, grape juice.

Vegetables: the aster family (lettuce, chicory, endive, globe and Jerusalem artichoke, salsify, sunflower seed sprouts); the beet family (beetroot, spinach, Swiss chard); the pea family (peas, mangetout, sugar peas, broad beans, runner beans, French beans, pulses including dried beans, lentils, chickpeas, lima beans, and soya beans).

Herbs and spices: tarragon, fenugreek seeds, nutmeg, liquorice, senna, red clover.

Fruit: peach, plum, apricot, cherry, nectarine, prune, cape gooseberries, dates, grapes, raisins.

Oils, etc.: sunflower, safflower, soya and almond oils (tropical oils – coconut or palm oil if available), wine vinegar, Balsamic vinegar.

the allergy exclusion diet

Suggested menus

Breakfasts

Fresh fruit salad

Compote of apricots and peaches

Rice porridge with prunes or Hunza apricots (p.83)

Rice pancakes with apricot or plum purée (p.87)

Rice flake muesli (p.84)

Soups and starters

Spinach and egg drop soup (p.110)

Green pea soup (p.110)

Bean sprouts and noodle soup (p.108)

Stuffed vine leaves (p.115)

Spinach and tofu puffs (p.121)

Almond and date stuffed peaches (p.120)

Chicken liver pâté (p.112)

Main meal dishes

Turkey and apricot pilaff (p.127)

Stir-fry duck with mangetout (p.127)

Pot roast pheasant/wild game bird (p.133)

Chicken with beetroot (p.126)

Roast chicken with plum stuffing (p.124)

Pigeon with prunes (p.132)

Vegetarian main meals

Artichoke and three-bean casserole (p.182)

Spinach and lentil flan (p.172)

Tempeh or tofu stir-fry (p.166)

Aduki bean burgers (p.163)

Spinach roulade with chickpea and salsify filling (p.183)

Apricot and almond pilaff (p.166)

Vegetables and salads

Cherry and almond salad (p.207)

Green bean salad (p.205)
Roasted Jerusalem artichokes (p.188)
Egg/tofu mayonnaise (p.195)

Puddings and desserts
Damson syllabub (p.227)
Chicory coffee ice cream (p.225)
Apricot and almond flan (p.228)

Cakes and biscuits
Sticky prune cake (p.216)
Rich fruit cake (p.215)
Carob and coconut brownies (p.217)
Cherry and coconut slices (p.221)
Rice bread (p.209)
Raisin bun loaf (p.209)

Drinks and miscellaneous
Rice milk (p.234)
Hot chocolate (p.235)
Soya milk (p.236)
Honey egg nog (p.236)
Almond and sunflower seed butters (p.238)

Day 4
The following foods can be eaten:
Cereals: buckwheat, buckwheat flour, buckwheat flakes and
buckwheat pasta, sweet potato flour, chestnut flour, tapioca,
amaranth, amaranth flour and amaranth pasta.
Meat, etc.: beef, lamb, sheep's milk product, goat's milk products,
cheese, butter, ghee, saltwater fish (cod, tuna, mackerel, eel, halibut,
plaice, anchovy, sole, sardine, hake, haddock).
Nuts & seeds: hazelnuts and spread, walnuts, pecan nuts,
chestnuts, poppy seeds, mustard seeds.
Sugars: maple syrup, apple and pear concentrate.

Drinks: sheep's milk, goat's milk, coffee, apple/pear juice, raspberry juice, raspberry leaf tea, rose-hip tea Equisetum tea, lemongrass tea.

Vegetables: the mustard family (Chinese leaves, cabbage, watercress, salad mustard and cress, mustard seed, cauliflower, broccoli, turnip, radish, horseradish, sprouts, kale, kohlrabi, swede); sweet potato; yam; dasheen, eddoes; sorrel.

Herbs and spices: the myrtle family (cloves, allspice), mustard seeds, lemongrass, capers.

Fruit: pear, apple, loquat, quince, lychees, the rose family (strawberry, raspberry, blackberry, rose-hip), pectin, rhubarb, guava.

Oils, etc.: hazelnut oil, walnut oil, cider vinegar, raspberry vinegar.

Suggested menus

Breakfasts

Buckwheat and amaranth porridge (p.83)

Buckwheat muesli (p.85)

Amaranth and apple pancakes (p.88)

Compote of strawberries and rhubarb

Soups and starters

Turnip and watercress soup (p.94)

Kohlrabi and goat's cheese soup (p.107)

Oxtail soup (p.109)

Pears with stilton (p.122)

Tuna fish roll (p.123)

Sprout and chestnut dip (p.117)

Lamb's liver with raspberries (p.120)

Main meal dishes

Fillet of beef with caper sauce (p.142)

Pot roast brisket of beef with horseradish sauce (p.143)

Lamb burgers (p.136)

Buckwheat and walnut coated herrings (p.155)

Grilled halibut with anchovy butter (p.155)

Fisherman's pie (p.154)

Vegetarian main meals

Feta cheese and cabbage pie (p.173)

Buckwheat pasta with broccoli and walnuts (p.176)

Buckwheat chappatis (p.212)

Vegetables and salads

Horseradish sauce (p.197)

Mustard sauce (p.194)

Fresh green salad (p.198)

Fresh winter salad (p.198)

Pear and watercress salad (p.207)

Baked red cabbage (p.190)

Bubble and squeak nests (p.192)

Puddings and desserts

Tapioca milk pudding (p.227)

Steamed apple pudding (p.229)

Bramble mouse (p.229)

Pears in raspberry sauce (p.230)

Cakes and biscuits

Buckwheat and chestnut dropped scones (p.220)

Apple and hazelnut muffins (p.219)

Drinks and miscellaneous

Strawberry yoghurt crush (p.232)

Rose hip cordial (p.232)

Hazelnut, walnut or pecan nut butter (p.239)

chapter 6 the recipes

BREAKFAST

Quinoa porridge

Good for: Preliminary Diet; Elimination Diet, Days 6, 8 &10;
Rotation Diet, Day 3
Serves 1
75 g quinoa (preferably soaked overnight)
450 ml mineral water

Place the quinoa in a saucepan and add the mineral water. Bring
to the boil and simmer for 20 to 30 minutes, or until well cooked.
NB: Millet porridge (see page 39) can be made in the same way,
replacing the quinoa with millet.

Speedy oat porridge

Good for: Rotation Diet, Day 2
Serves 2
100 g organic rolled oatflakes
1 litre water

Place the oats in a saucepan and add the cold water. Bring to the
boil and simmer for 1 minute, stirring as it thickens.

Sorghum porridge

Good for: Elimination Diet, Day 8; Rotation Diet, Day 2

Serves 2

100 g sorghum meal

1 litre water

pinch of salt

Cook as for the speedy oat porridge, stirring all the time.

Millet and kamut porridge

Good for: Elimination Diet, Day 11; Rotation Diet, Day 1

Serves 2

75 g millet flakes

25 g kamut, soaked overnight

500 ml water

Place the grains and flakes in a saucepan and add the water. Bring to the boil and simmer for 4 to 5 minutes until the kamut is soft and the porridge thickens. Serve with barley malt, chopped figs or cashew nut milk.

Old-fashioned oatmeal porridge

Good for: Elimination Diet, Day 16; Rotation Diet, Day 2

Serves 2 to 3

100 g pinhead oatmeal or whole oat groats

1 litre water

pinch of salt

Place the oats in a saucepan (double boiler if available), add the cold water and salt and bring to the boil. Turn off the heat and leave overnight. Next morning, bring to the boil again and simmer for 30 minutes, stirring from time to time.

Buckwheat and amaranth porridge

Good for: Rotation Diet, Day 4

Serves 2 to 3

50 g amaranth, soaked overnight

125 g buckwheat flakes

1 litre water

pinch of sea salt

Place the grains and flakes in a saucepan and add the water and salt. Bring to the boil and simmer gently for about 5 minutes until the amaranth is soft and the porridge thickens, stirring occasionally.

Rice porridge with prunes or hunza apricots

Good for: Elimination Diet, Day 12; Rotation Diet, Day 3

Serves 4

200 g organic short wholegrain rice

2 litres water

prunes or hunza apricots

Bring all the ingredients to the boil, then simmer very gently for a good hour until all the water has been absorbed. Cooking the rice in this way, helps to preserve the nutrients and makes a very digestible and cleansing food for the gut.

Hunza apricots are the best and are available at some health food stores or may be ordered. Soak overnight and then cook for 7 to 10 minutes. Once soaked, the hunza apricots may also be eaten uncooked. The kernels can be cracked open and eaten as nuts. Prepare prunes in the same way as the apricots. Buy prunes and apricots from health food stores and avoid the 'ready-to-eat, no need to soak' preparations.

Barley flake muesli

Good for: Rotation Diet, Day 1

Serves 4

200 g barley flakes or a mixture of flakes from wheat, rye or millet grains

cashew nuts

ground linseeds

sesame seeds

chopped dried or fresh figs

mango

Mix together all the ingredients and serve with mango or orange juice or cashew nut milk.

Rice flake muesli

Good for: Preliminary Diet; Rotation Diet, Day 3

Serves 4

rice flakes

chopped nuts

dried fruit or top with fresh fruit

soya, rice or nut milks

Soak the rice flakes in liquid for 5 to 10 minutes before serving. Mix together all the ingredients and serve with mango or orange juice, cashew nut milk or with grape juice or the juice left over from cooking prunes and apricots.

Oat flake muesli

Good for: Rotation Diet, Day 2

Serves 4

200 g jumbo oatflakes

50 g oat bran and germ (optional)

chopped Brazil nuts

pumpkins seeds

fresh or sun dried bananas

Mix together all the ingredients and serve with pineapple juice, stewed gooseberries or tiger nut milk.

Buckwheat muesli

Good for: Elimination Diet, Days 7 & 15; Rotation Diet, Day 4

Serves 4

225 g buckwheat flakes

50 g flaked or whole hazelnuts

50 g pecan nut pieces

fresh or dried fruit, e.g. apple, pear, raspberries, chopped

sheep's milk, rice milk or permitted fruit juice

rice syrup or maple syrup (optional)

Mix together all the dry ingredients and leave to soak with the milk or fruit juice for 5 to 7 minutes to soften. If you choose, serve with rice syrup or maple syrup.

Polenta (maize meal)

Good for: Elimination Diet, Day 16; Rotation Diet, Day 2

Serves 4

600 ml water

1 tsp sea salt

225 g fine maize meal (polenta)

In a heavy-based saucepan, bring the water to the boil with the salt and gradually add the maize meal, stirring with a wooden spoon to keep it smooth. Cook gently for 20 minutes until it thickens and comes cleanly away from the sides of the pan.

Pour into a well oiled, shallow baking dish, approximately 20 x 31 cm. Spread out with a wet spatula so the polenta is roughly 1-cm thick.

Frumenty

Good for: Rotation Diet, Day 1

Serves 4

225 g organic whole wheat grains

1 litre water

Wash the wheat grains and pre-soak for 6 to 8 hours. Place in a pan with the remaining water and bring to the boil. Simmer gently for 10 minutes and then leave in a warm place overnight.

At the end, of this time, the wheat grains should have burst open and look starchy and white and form a thick jelly. If some are still whole, boil up again and cook gently for a little while longer. Serve with fruit for breakfast or supper.

Barley/rice and sesame seed snacks

Good for: Elimination Diet, Day 12

Serves 4

125 g barley or rice flour

1 tbsp sago or tapioca flour

250 ml water

2 tbsp tahini

1 tbsp sesame seeds

2 tbsp sesame seed oil

1 to 2 tbsp honey

Preheat the oven to 150°C/Gas mark 2.

Mix together all the ingredients with enough water to make a piping consistency. Beat well and place in a piping bag, fitted with a large nozzle and pipe out shapes onto a lined baking tray. Bake for 30 minutes.

Savoury snacks can be made by substituting the honey and cinnamon with ½ tsp cardamom, 1 tsp of dried herbs and a pinch of salt.

Rice pancakes with apricot or plum purée

Good for: Rotation Diet, Day 3

Serves 4

125 g rice flour

1 egg

1 tsp cream of tartar

250 ml soya or coconut milk

Place all the ingredients in a liquidiser and blend well, adding more liquid if necessary. Dry fry on a griddle or in a heavy-based pan and pour in sufficient batter to make 1 pancake at a time. Cook until just golden on both sides and keep warm. Serve with apricot or plum purée and sweeten with honey if needed.

Waffles and drop scones may be made with this batter mixture using less liquid.

Amaranth and apple pancakes

Good for: Rotation Diet, Day 4

Serves 4

FOR THE BATTER

125 g amaranth flour

1 tsp cream of tartar

½ tsp bicarbonate of soda

125 ml water or sheep's milk

½ tsp allspice

1 to 2 dessert apples

Mix together the ingredients for the batter and beat well adding more liquid if necessary to form a pouring consistency.

Peel and cut the apple into quarters and then into fine slices. Pour a little at a time of the pancake mixture onto a hot, non-stick griddle or pan to make individual pancakes. Cook for 1 minute and then add some slices of apple to the pancake so the apple sinks in but not to the bottom. Turn and cook for a further minute on the other side. Roll up and serve.

Pear and ginger fruit slice

Good for: Elimination Diet, Day 14

Serves 4

4 quail's eggs (optional)

2 pears, peeled, cored and thinly sliced

125 g barley flour

125 g ground almonds

125 ml sesame seed oil

2 tbsp honey to taste

1 tsp ground ginger

1 tsp grated lemon zest

Preheat the oven to 150°C/Gas mark 2.

Beat the eggs and mix in the other ingredients. Spoon into a well-oiled baking tin and cook for 30 to 35 minutes.

Avocado fruit cocktail

Good for: Elimination Diet, Day 27

Serves 4

2 peaches, skinned and chopped

125 ml water

juice of 1 lemon

2 tbsp maple syrup

2 avocado pears, peeled and sliced

125 g green seedless grapes

125 g strawberries

Cook the peaches in the water for 2 to 3 minutes until just soft and allow to cool. Strain off the juice and mix this with the lemon juice and maple syrup. Divide the peach pieces between 4 individual glass bowls and arrange the rest of the fruit on top and pour over the juice.

Vegetable hash browns

Good for: Preliminary Diet; Elimination Diet, Day 5

Serves 4

225 g turnip or swede, peeled, cooked and mashed

125 g finely sliced and chopped white cabbage

125 g brown rice flour

sea salt

Preheat the oven to 160°C/Gas mark 3.

Mix together all the ingredients and shape into cakes. Place on a baking tray and cook for 20 minutes. These may be made up in larger quantities for freezing.

Grilled trout

Good for: Rotation Diet, Day 1

Serves 4

4 medium sized river trout

sea salt or kelp

1 tbsp fresh dill, chopped or 1 tsp dried

1 tbsp sesame seeds

Place the trout in a grill pan. Make two or three slashes across the skin and sprinkle with salt or kelp. Grill on one side only for 5 to 7 minutes until just cooked through. There should be no need to turn. Sprinkle with dill and sesame seeds and serve.

SOUPS AND STARTERS

Vegetable stock (potassium broth)
Good for: Preliminary Diet
Serves 4

Use vegetables, seaweeds and trimmings but note that too many mustard family greens or spinach may spoil the flavour. Simmer gently, with plenty of water and with the lid on the saucepan for 1½ to 2 hours. The nutrients will leach into the stock, which can then be strained off and the fibre remains discarded. Take great care to label containers with all the ingredients, particularly if you are freezing the stock and when checking your allergies.

Lamb stock
Good for: Preliminary Diet
Serves 4

Use raw bones from organically reared mutton or lamb, chopped into 5-cm pieces. Wash and place in a large, heavy saucepan or pressure cooker. Cover with cold water and a pinch of salt and bring to the boil. Simmer for 3 hours or for 1½ hours in a pressure cooker. Strain the stock and allow to cool. Skim off the fat before use.

The stock may be frozen in an ice-cube tray or kept in a refrigerator for up to 2 days.

Poultry or game stock
Good for: Rotation Diet, Day 3
Serves 4

Turkey, duck, goose, chicken or game stock can be made from the carcass, giblets, skin and legs of the bird. Cook for 1½ hours (45 minutes in a pressure cooker), strain, allow to cool and skim off the fat.

Fish stock

Good for: Preliminary Diet

Serves 4

Wash the trimmings and break up the bones. Cover with cold water, add a little sea salt and bring to simmering point. Cook gently for no longer than 30 minutes to avoid bitterness. Use or freeze.

Cream of cauliflower soup with almonds

Good for: Preliminary Diet; Rotation Diet, Day 3

Serves 4

1 litre mineral water or stock
1 small sweet potato, peeled and roughly chopped
1 small cauliflower
3 sticks celery
sea salt
125 g ground almonds

Bring the water to the boil. Add the sweet potato, cauliflower and celery and a pinch of salt. Cook for 5 to 7 minutes until the vegetables are tender.

Allow to cool slightly. Take out a few cauliflower florets. Add the ground almonds and liquidise until smooth. Return to the pan. Add the cauliflower florets and reheat gently.

the allergy exclusion diet

Celery and courgette soup

Good for: Preliminary Diet

Serves 4

1 litre stock or mineral water

6 sticks celery, diced

2 courgettes, cut lengthways and sliced

1 small sweet potato or yam, diced

sea salt or kelp

fresh coriander leaves, chopped

Bring the stock/water to the boil and add the vegetables and season. Cover and cook for 10 minutes until the vegetables are tender. Ladle out half the vegetables and liquidise to a purée. Return to the pan, reheat and serve with a garnishing of coriander or other fresh herb.

Celery and chestnut soup

Good for: Preliminary Diet

Serves 4

125 g dried chestnuts, soaked

1 litre stock or mineral water

1 bunch of celery, roughly sliced

1 bay leaf

sea salt

freshly chopped parsley

Cook the chestnuts in half the water for 1 hour. Meanwhile steam the celery or gently sauté in olive oil, reserving 1 or 2 finely diced sticks for garnishing. Cool slightly and liquidise to a purée with the chestnuts. Add the remaining stock or water and bay leaf and some salt. Reheat and serve with the diced celery and parsley.

Green split pea soup with broccoli

Good for: Preliminary Diet

Serves 4

125 g green split peas
1 litre stock and/or mineral water
2 bay leaves
½ tsp dried marjoram
½ tsp lemongrass
1 tsp salt
450 g broccoli, chopped
125 g broccoli florets

Pre-soak the split peas in hot water for 1 to 2 hours (they will not sprout). Place in a pan with the water, bay leaves, herbs and seasoning and cook for about 30 minutes until tender. Add the chopped broccoli and any remaining stock and cook for a further 10 minutes. Remove the bay leaves and leave to cool slightly. Liquidise until smooth and return to the pan to reheat.

Meanwhile, steam the broccoli florets in a little water until tender but still green and add to the soup

Turnip and watercress soup

Good for: Elimination Diet, Day 5; can be adapted for Rotation Day 4 by adding yoghurt or cheese

Serves 4

1 bunch watercress
1 litre lamb stock and/or mineral water
450 g turnips, peeled and roughly chopped
sea salt

Wash the watercress and separate the stalks from the leaves. Bring the stock/water to the boil and add the turnips. Simmer until tender. Liquidise with the watercress stalks and return to the pan. Add seasoning and the sprigs of watercress and cook for a further minute.

the allergy exclusion diet

Cream of carrot and celeriac soup

Good for: Preliminary Diet; Elimination Diet, Day 7

Serves 4

275 g carrots, chopped

275 g celeriac, chopped

1 litre mineral water, game stock or parsley family stock

sea salt

2 tbsp olive oil

2 tbsp chopped parsley or coriander leaves, for garnishing

Cook the vegetables in some of the stock/water, until tender. Liquidise until smooth and creamy. Return to the pan, add seasoning and the remaining liquid and reheat. Cook for a further 2 minutes, add the oil and serve with a garnishing of chopped parsley.

Yam and chicory soup

Good for: Elimination Diet, Day 8

Serves 4

500 ml mineral water/stock

225 g yam, peeled and chopped

sea salt

2 heads of chicory, chopped

1 tbsp fresh tarragon, chopped, for garnishing

Bring the water to the boil. Add the yam and a pinch of salt. Bring to the boil and simmer until tender. Liquidise and return to the pan. Add the chicory and cook for 1 minute. Sprinkle with tarragon and serve.

Swiss chard and celery soup

Good for: Elimination Diet, Day 10

Serves 4

4 sticks celery

350 g Swiss chard or spinach

125 g sweet potato or yam

1 litre stock or water

sea salt

fresh thyme or ½ tsp dried

Reserve a celery stick and a leaf of Swiss chard. Roughly chop the remaining vegetables and boil in a little water, in order of cooking time. Blend in a liquidiser and return to the saucepan with the stock/water and bring to the boil. Season with salt and thyme and add the reserved leaf of Swiss chard cut into slithers and the celery stick thinly sliced. Cook for a further 2 minutes.

Onion and barley soup

Good for: Elimination Diet, Day 15

Serves 4

450 g onions thinly sliced

125 g pot barley

1 bay leaf

1 litre game or vegetable stock or water

arame seaweed, washed and soaked

olive oil

1 tbsp tamari soya sauce

chopped parsley, for garnishing

Place the onions, barley and bay leaf in a pan and cover with half the water/stock. Cook for 20 minutes until the barley is soft. Add the arame seaweed and soaking water and the remaining stock and bring to boiling point. Simmer for a further 10 minutes. Stir in the olive oil and tamari sauce and garnish with chopped parsley.

the allergy exclusion diet

Cream of asparagus soup

Good for: Elimination Diet, Day 11

Serves 4

450 g asparagus

1 large onion

1 litre game or vegetable stock or water

50 g ground almonds

sea salt

juice of 1 lemon

1 tbsp fresh parsley, chopped, for garnishing

Wash and prepare the asparagus. Cut off the tips and trim off the coarse outer parts of the remaining stems. Cut into 2-cm pieces. Cook the tips in a little water and drain, reserving the water. The tips are not needed in this recipe.

Cook the onion and the asparagus stems in the water for 5 to 7 minutes until soft. Make up the quantity of liquid with the stock/water and add the ground almonds and salt. Liquidise the soup to a creamy constituency and serve with chopped parsley. Serve with the lemon juice and a garnishing of chopped parsley.

Baked tomato soup

Good for: Elimination Diet, Day 12; Rotation Diet, Day 2

Serves 4

750 g tomatoes,

1 onion, sliced

2 cloves garlic

1 litre pork stock or water

2 tbsp freshly chopped basil

sea salt

Preheat the oven to 180°C/Gas mark 4. Cut the tomatoes into halves and scoop out the seeds. Place on a baking tray with the onion and garlic cloves and bake for 20 minutes. Remove from the oven and take the skins off the tomatoes. Cool slightly and then liquidise.

Bring the stock/water to the boil and add the baked ingredients together with the basil and salt. Cook for 5 minutes and serve with a sprinkling of basil.

Miso soup

Good for: Elimination Diet, Day 16

Serves 4

1 carrot, diced

½ small cauliflower, broken into florets

50 g peas

4 spring onions sliced

1 clove garlic, crushed

1 tsp grated ginger

1 litre water

1 tbsp miso soya bean paste

2 sheets nori seaweed cut into 2.5-cm squares

Gently cook the vegetables and seasonings in the water until soft. Blend the miso in a little of the soup liquid and add to the soup but do not allow to boil. Add the nori and serve.

Yellow split pea soup

Good for: Elimination Diet, Day 13

Serves 4

125 g yellow split peas, soaked

1 litre stock or water

1 tsp caraway seeds

1 bay leaf

sea salt

3 sticks celery, chopped

175 g yam or sweet potato, diced

2 tbsp olive oil

parsley, for garnishing

Allow the split peas to soak in hot water for 1 to 2 hours (these have been processed and will not sprout). Cook the peas, gently with the seasoning, for 40 minutes until beginning to turn mushy. Remove the bay leaf.

Cook the celery and potatoes in some of the water/stock until soft. Add to the split peas and liquidise until smooth. Return to the pan, add the remaining liquid and reheat. Cook for 2 minutes. Stir in the olive oil and serve with a garnishing of chopped parsley.

Mushroom and black bean soup

Good for: Elimination Diet, Day 17

Serves 4

2 leeks, thinly sliced

1 litre stock or water

125 g wild mushrooms, diced

125 g black beans, soaked, sprouted and cooked

1 tbsp soya, gram or barley flour

1 bay leaf

sprig of thyme

Cook the leeks until tender. Add the stock/water and bring to the boil. Mix in the mushrooms, beans and seasoning and cook gently for 15 to 20 minutes. Remove the bay leaf and thyme and serve.

Leek and potato soup

Good for: Elimination Diet, Day 20

Serves 4

450 g potatoes, peeled and diced

3 leeks, sliced

2 bay leaves

sprig of rosemary

1 litre stock or water

sea salt

bunch of chives, chopped

creamed sheep's cheese or yoghurt (optional)

Gently cook the vegetables, bay leaves and rosemary in some of the stock/water for 20 minutes. Remove the rosemary and bay leaves. Allow to cool slightly and blend in a liquidiser. Add the salt and chopped chives and reheat gently. May be served with sheep's cheese or yoghurt.

Garden vegetable soup

Good for: Elimination Diet, Day 23

Serves 4

1 litre stock or water

175 g small pickling onions

175 g broccoli florets

2 carrots, thinly sliced

2 courgettes, diced

125 g button mushrooms, quartered

1 tbsp barley or gram flour

sea salt or kelp

fresh thyme, for garnishing

Pour the stock/water into a saucepan and bring to the boil. Add all the ingredients, bring to the boiling and simmer until cooked.

Cream of artichoke soup

Good for: Elimination Diet, Day 24

Serves 4

1 litre chicken, game or vegetable stock

675 g Jerusalem artichokes, peeled and sliced

1 large onion, sliced

pinch of nutmeg

125 ml goat's milk yoghurt

sprigs of watercress or freshly chopped tarragon, for garnishing

Pour the stock into a saucepan and bring to the boil. Add the artichokes, onion and seasoning and return to the boil. Cover and simmer for 20 minutes until all the vegetables are tender. Cool slightly and liquidise until smooth. Re-heat and serve with goat's milk yoghurt and a garnishing of watercress or tarragon.

Chicken noodle main meal soup

Good for: Elimination Diet, Day 27

Serves 4

600 ml water or stock

225 g free-range chicken breast

125 g fresh peas

4 spring onions sliced

2 carrots, diced

1 tsp grated ginger

1 tsp ground coriander

½ tsp ground turmeric

sea salt or kelp

250 ml coconut milk

175 g rice noodles

coriander leaves, for garnishing

Pour the water/stock into a saucepan and bring to the boil. Cut the chicken into thin strips and add to the pan to seal. Add the vegetables and spices and bring to the boil. Cover and simmer for 35 minutes. Add the coconut milk and noodles and simmer, stirring for another 5 to 8 minutes. Garnish with chopped coriander leaves and serve.

Minestrone soup

Good for: Elimination Diet, Day 28

Serves 4

1 litre stock

1 potato, diced

2 carrots, cut in half lengthways and thinly sliced

2 bay leaves

450 g tomatoes, skinned and diced

125 g green beans, cut into short pieces

1 courgette, diced

2 onions, chopped

2 cloves garlic, crushed

sea salt

50 g white cabbage, shredded

2 tbsp fresh basil or oregano, chopped

125 g flageolet beans, sprouted and cooked

125 g wholemeal pasta shapes (wheat, barley, millet or rice), cooked

grated Parmesan cheese (optional)

Pour the stock into a pan and bring to the boil and add the potato, carrots, bay leaves and the remaining vegetables in order of cooking time and season. Simmer for 20 minutes and then add the shredded cabbage, basil, flageolet beans and pasta and cook for a further 2 to 3 minutes. Remove the bay leaves and serve with Parmesan cheese.

Avocado and green pepper soup

Good for: Rotation Diet, Day 2

Serves 4

2 green peppers, deseeded and chopped

1 litre stock or water

2 bay leaves

sea salt

2 large avocado pears

freshly chopped mint, for garnishing

Cook the peppers in a little of the stock/water with the bay leaves and a pinch of salt until tender. Remove the bay leaves.

Peel and stone the avocado and place the flesh in a liquidiser and pour in the contents of the saucepan. Blend to a purée and return to the saucepan to reheat adding the remaining stock. Serve with a sprinkling of chopped mint.

Spiced pumpkin and ginger soup

Good for: Elimination Diet, Day 22; Rotation Diet, Day 2

Serves 4

900 g pumpkin or squash flesh, diced

1 tsp root ginger, grated

2 cloves garlic, crushed

1 dried chilli, crushed

1 tsp ground turmeric

sea salt

1 litre stock or water

Place all the ingredients in a large saucepan. Cover with some of the water/stock and bring to the boil. Simmer for 10 minutes and allow to cool slightly. Place in a liquidiser and blend until smooth. Return to the saucepan, adding the remaining stock and cook for a further 5 minutes.

Parsnip and coriander soup

Good for: Rotation Diet, Day 1

Serves 4

1 litre vegetable stock

675 g parsnips, diced

2 sticks celery, sliced

sea salt or kelp

½ tsp ground coriander

½ tsp ground cumin

2 tbsp fresh coriander leaves, chopped, for garnishing

Place half the stock in a saucepan and bring to the boil. Add the parsnips, celery, salt or kelp and ground spices and cook until tender. Cool slightly and then liquidise to a purée. Return to the pan with the remaining stock and reheat. Serve with a garnishing of fresh coriander.

Mushroom and barley broth

Good for: Rotation Diet, Day 1

Serves 4

225 g mushrooms, diced

175 g pot barley

2 carrots, diced

1 litre stock or water

sea salt or 1 tsp barley miso

2 tbsp chopped parsley, for garnishing

Put all the ingredients into a casserole dish, bring to the boil, cover with a lid and simmer gently for 40 to 50 minutes until the barley is cooked, adding more liquid if necessary. Serve with a sprinkling of chopped parsley.

Clear vegetable and nori broth

Good for: Rotation Diet, Day 1

Serves 4

1 litre vegetable, lamb or fish stock or water

2 large carrots, cut into matchsticks

2 sticks celery, thinly sliced

1 small parsnip, diced

1 tsp barley miso, sea salt, kelp

2 to 3 sheets nori seaweed, cut into 2.5-cm squares

1 tbsp sesame seed oil

Place some of the water/stock in a pan and bring to the boil. Add the vegetables and cook until tender. Add the remaining stock, miso and nori seaweed, bring to the boil and simmer for 1 minute. Stir in the sesame seed oil and serve.

Fish and fennel soup

Good for: Rotation Diet, Day 1

Serves 4

1 litre fish or vegetable stock or water

1 head of fennel, cut into strips

2 carrots, diced

1 tsp dried fennel

sea salt or 1 tsp kelp

125 g freshwater fish, filleted

125 g mixed shellfish, shelled

50 g small pasta shells

2 tbsp fresh parsley, chopped

Bring some of the stock/water to the boil and cook the fennel and carrots until just tender. Add the remaining liquid, dried fennel and salt or kelp and re-boil. Add the fish and pasta and cook for another 5 minutes, adding the parsley during the last minute of cooking. Cook the pasta separately if a larger, longer cooking variety is used.

Kohlrabi and goat's cheese soup

Good for: Rotation Diet, Day 4

Serves 4

450 g kohlrabi, diced

1 small sweet potato, diced

1 litre stock or water

125 g soft goat's cheese

½ tsp allspice

sea salt

salad cress, for garnishing

Cook the kohlrabi and sweet potato in the stock/water until tender. Remove the rind from the goat's cheese and liquidise with the vegetables. Add the seasoning and re-heat. Serve with a sprinkling of chopped salad cress.

Sweetcorn and lima bean succotash soup

Good for: Elimination Diet, Day 18

Serves 4

125 g yam, diced

125 g courgette, diced

2 sticks celery, sliced

250 ml vegetable stock or water

175 g lima beans, sprouted and cooked

350 g sweetcorn kernels

1 sprig thyme

3 sage leaves, chopped

2 tbsp olive oil

sea salt

Cook the yam, courgette and celery in the stock/water for 5 to 7 minutes in order of cooking time. Add the remaining ingredients and simmer for 10 minutes.

Lentil soup

Good for: Preliminary Diet; Elimination Diet, Day 9

Serves 4

1 litre water or stock

125 g brown lentils, pre-soaked

2 large carrots, roughly chopped

1 parsnip, roughly chopped

2 sticks celery, roughly chopped

1 tsp cumin seeds

sea salt

1 tbsp chopped coriander leaves, for garnishing

Bring the water/stock to the boil. Add the lentils, vegetables, cumin seeds and salt. Simmer gently until the vegetables are tender. Liquidise and return to the pan to reheat. Serve with a sprinkling of fresh coriander leaves.

Bean sprouts and noodle soup

Good for: Rotation Diet, Day 3

Serves 4

125 g chickpea sprouts

125 g lentil sprouts

125 g mung bean sprouts

1 litre water

3 stalks Swiss chard, sliced

1 to 2 tsp miso or sea salt

50 g rice noodles

Chop the chickpeas and place in a large saucepan together with the lentil and mung bean sprouts and cover with boiling water. Cook for 10 to 15 minutes until tender. Add the Swiss chard, miso or salt and rice noodles and cook for a further 7 to 10 minutes.

Gazpacho

Good for: Rotation Diet, Day 2

Serves 4

450 g tomatoes peeled, deseeded and chopped

250 ml stock or water

4 tbsp olive oil

2 onions, chopped

1 large cucumber, peeled and diced

1 large green pepper, deseeded and diced

2 cloves garlic, crushed

black pepper

Blend half the tomatoes, stock and olive oil to a purée. Mix in with the vegetables and refrigerate for 2 to 4 hours before serving.

Oxtail soup

Good for: Rotation Diet, Day 4

Serves 4

2 small oxtails from organically reared beef

1 litre water

2 small turnips, halved and sliced

125 g swede, diced

1 tsp mustard seeds

sea salt

1 tbsp tapioca flour

Wash and dry the oxtails and cut into joints. Put the water in a saucepan and bring to the boil. Add the oxtail joints, vegetables and seasoning and return to the boil. Simmer gently for 3 hours or pressure cook for 1½ hours. Take out the pieces of oxtail and cut the meat from the bone. Return the meat to the soup and re-heat. Mix the tapioca flour with a little cold water and stir into the soup.

There may be some fat on the soup, which can be removed with a basting pipette or allow to cool overnight and skim the fat from the top.

Green pea soup

Good for: Rotation Diet, Day 3

Serves 4

450 g fresh peas in their pods

1 cos lettuce

1 litre water

sea salt

125 ml soya cream

Shell the peas and reserve the pods. Take the outer leaves from the lettuce and cook with the pods for 10 minutes in some of the water. Cool a little and liquidise to a purée. Pour through a sieve and discard the pulp.

Place the stock to one side and bring the remaining water to the boil. Add the peas, sliced lettuce leaves and salt and cook for 7 to 10 minutes. Liquidise and return to the pan with the pea stock. Reheat and stir in the soya cream, if using, before serving.

This soup may also be served with shredded smoked tofu instead of soya cream.

Spinach and egg drop soup

Good for: Rotation Diet, Day 3

Serves 4

225 g spinach, washed and chopped

1 litre chicken stock or water

½ tsp nutmeg

2 tsp miso or sea salt

2 eggs, lightly beaten

Place the spinach in a saucepan and cover with boiling stock/water. Cook for 3 to 4 minutes until tender. Cool slightly, then liquidise to a purée. Return to the pan, add the remaining stock/water, nutmeg and seasoning and reheat. Remove from the heat and add the eggs, stirring until they separate into strands. Serve immediately.

Pistachio and rabbit pâté

Good for: Rotation Diet, Day 1

Serves 4

1 tbsp sesame seed oil

450 g boneless rabbit meat and/or rabbit livers

125 g celeriac, diced

225 ml water or stock

2 tbsp chopped parsley

1 rounded tbsp barley or wheat flour

75 g pistachio nuts, chopped

sea salt

black pepper

Warm the sesame seed oil and a little water in a pan and gently cook the rabbit meat on both sides for 4 to 5 minutes. Put to one side and cook the celeriac in the juices until soft. Add the water/stock and parsley and bring to the boil. Simmer for 2 to 3 minutes. Mix the flour with a little cold water and stir into the liquid, to make a thick sauce. Cool slightly and liquidise with the meat to make a smooth paste. Turn into a bowl and stir in the pistachio nuts, salt and pepper and serve chilled with bread or crackers.

Chicken liver pâté

Good for: Rotation Diet, Day 3

Serves 4

FOR THE WHITE SAUCE

1 tbsp rice flour

225 ml soya/nut milk or stock (or a mixture)

FOR THE PÂTÉ

4 chicken livers

1 tbsp dripping

250 ml thick white sauce

1 egg

1 tbsp freshly chopped tarragon

pinch of nutmeg

sea salt

To make the white sauce, mix the rice flour with a little water. Bring the milk/stock to the boil and stir in the rice flour. Cook until the sauce thickens.

For the pâté, wash and trim the livers. Heat the dripping in a pan and cook the livers gently until just cooked. Cool slightly and place in a food processor with the white sauce and the remaining ingredients. Blend until smooth and turn into a pâté dish and refrigerate.

Stuffed mushrooms

Good for: Preliminary Diet; Elimination Diet, Day 21; Rotation
 Diet, Day 1

Serves 4

8 large flat mushrooms
300 g cooked millet or 100 g millet cooked in 300 ml water
1 tbsp tahini
2 tbsp fresh coriander, chopped
sea salt
1 tbsp sesame seeds
lemon wedges, for serving

Preheat the oven to 160°C/Gas mark 3.

Peel the mushrooms and remove the stalks. Chop the stalks and place in a bowl and mix with the millet, tahini, coriander and salt. Place the mixture on the mushrooms and sprinkle with sesame seeds. Bake for 20 minutes until the mushrooms are cooked and the stuffing crisp. Serve with lemon wedges.

Stuffed tomatoes

Good for: Elimination Diet, Day 19

Serves 4

4 large tomatoes

125 g quinoa, cooked

50 g pumpkin seeds, dry roasted and chopped

50 g Brazil nuts, finely chopped

1 large onion, chopped and fried

1 clove garlic, crushed

1 tbsp freshly chopped herbs e.g. basil, thyme or marjoram

sea salt

Preheat the oven to 160°C/Gas mark 3.

Cut the tops off the tomatoes and scoop out all the flesh. Discard the seeds and chop the remainder. Make a mixture with the remaining ingredients and spoon back into the tomato shells. Bake for 20 minutes.

This stuffing may also be used for stuffing marrow, courgette, aubergine and peppers. The cooking time may vary.

Stuffed vine leaves

Good for: Rotation Diet, Day 3

Serves 4

FOR THE FILLING

125 g rice, cooked

125 g brown lentils, sprouted and cooked

25 g sprouted fenugreek seeds

125 g sunflower seeds, chopped

50 g raisins

nutmeg

sea salt

225 g vine leaves

sprigs of tarragon, for garnishing

Mix together all the ingredients for the filling. Spread out the vine leaves, smooth side down and place a tablespoonful of the mixture in the centre of the bottom edge of each leaf. Fold in the sides and roll up firmly to form a small sausage-shaped parcel. There should be enough filling for about 20 parcels (or dolmas).

Using a heavy-based shallow saucepan, line the bottom of the pan with the remaining vine leaves and closely pack the dolmas into the saucepan. Add sufficient water to cover and bring to the boil. Simmer gently for 1 minute, leave to cool and then drain. Garnish with the tarragon.

Spinach leaves may be used instead of vine leaves.

Tortillas with sweetcorn and tomato filling

Good for: Elimination Diet, Day 22; Rotation Diet, Day 2

Serves 4

FOR THE FILLING

1 onion, chopped

2 cloves garlic, crushed

4 tomatoes, skinned and chopped

225 g cooked sweetcorn

1 tbsp tomato purée

2 tsp fresh oregano

sea salt

FOR THE TORTILLAS

175 g maize flour

250 ml warm water

2 tbsp olive oil

½ tsp sea salt

For the filling, cook the onion and garlic in a little water until soft. Add the tomatoes and sweetcorn and cook for another 5 minutes. Mix with the tomato purée and seasoning.

For the tortillas, put the maize flour in a bowl and gradually beat in the water and oil. Knead until a smooth, elastic dough is formed. Divide into eight portions and roll out each one between two sheets of greaseproof paper or tough polythene to form a thin round about 15 cm in diameter. Dry fry or cook on a hot griddle for 2 to 3 minutes on each side. Spoon 2 to 3 tbsp of filling into each tortilla, fold over and keep warm on a serving dish.

Avocado may be used instead of sweetcorn.

Avocado and courgette dip

Good for: Rotation Diet, Day 2

Serves 4

2 large ripe avocado pears
125 g cooked courgette
2 cloves garlic, crushed
sea salt
paprika pepper

FOR THE CRUDITÉS

1 red, yellow and green pepper, deseeded and cut lengthways
1 cucumber, cut into 5-cm chunks and then cut lengthways
baby corn

Scoop out the flesh of the avocados and mash together with the cooked courgette. Add the seasoning and serve with crudités or tortillas.

Sprout and chestnut dip

Good for: Rotation Diet, Day 4

Serves 4

225 g Brussels sprouts
225 g cooked chestnuts
1 tsp ground lemongrass
sea salt

FOR THE CRUDITÉS

raw swede, cut into pieces
turnip or kohlrabi, cut into matchsticks
radishes, cauliflower florets, Chinese leaf stalks

Cook the Brussels sprouts in a little water for 3 to 4 minutes until soft. Cool slightly and liquidise with the chestnuts and seasoning. Blend to a smooth purée adding some of the cooking water if necessary. Allow to cool and serve with the crudités.

Hummus and cannellini bean dip

Good for: Elimination Diet, Day 16

Serves 4

225 g chickpeas, sprouted and cooked or 225 g cannellini beans, sprouted

4 tbsp tahini

juice of 2 lemons

2 cloves garlic

1 tbsp olive oil

1 tbsp sesame seed oil

black pepper, sea salt

parsley and paprika pepper or fresh mint and ground cumin, for garnishing

For the hummus, place the chickpeas and all the remaining ingredients in a food processor and mix until smooth using some of the chick pea cooking water if necessary. Serve with crudités – sticks of carrot, celery, green, red and yellow peppers, cauliflower florets, radishes, chicory leaves etc.

For the cannellini bean dip, follow the recipe for hummus using sprouted cannellini beans instead of chickpeas and flavour with chopped fresh mint and ground cumin. Garnish with a sprig of mint.

Tomato relish

Good for: Elimination Diet, Day 28

Serves 4

225 g tomatoes, skinned, seeded and chopped

4 spring onions, chopped

50 g capers

1 stick celery, chopped

paprika pepper

1 tbsp tomato purée

freshly chopped basil

pinch of allspice

sea salt

Mix together the ingredients and use as required.

Sweetcorn relish

Good for: Elimination Diet, Day 28

Serves 4

225 g sweetcorn

1 red pepper, deseeded and chopped

½ cucumber, diced

½ tsp chilli powder (optional)

½ tsp ground mustard

black pepper

sea salt

Place half the sweetcorn in a liquidiser and blend. Mix with the remaining ingredients.

Date and Apple chutney

Good for: Elimination Diet, Day 28

Serves 4

250 ml cider vinegar

225 g eating apples, chopped

225 g cooking apples, chopped

225 g stoned dates, chopped

225 g sultanas

225 g onions, chopped

125 g raw cane molasses sugar (optional)

1 tsp grated ginger

pinch of allspice

sea salt

Bring the vinegar to the boil and add all the ingredients. Cook for 15 to 20 minutes until tender and the cooking apples have become mushy. Keep refrigerated or may be bottled or frozen.

Lamb's liver with raspberries

Good for: Rotation Diet, Day 4

Serves 4

225 g raspberries

2 tsps maple syrup

2 tbsp raspberry vinegar

225 g lamb's liver

sea salt

Chinese leaves, for garnishing

Reserve 12 raspberries for garnishing and purée the remainder in a liquidiser. Strain and stir in the maple syrup and vinegar.

Cut the liver into thin strips, sprinkle with a little salt and grill for 3 to 4 minutes, turning until all sides are cooked. Arrange the liver on four warmed plates and pour over the raspberry sauce. Garnish with Chinese leaves.

Almond and date stuffed peaches

Good for: Rotation Diet, Day 3

Serves 4

2 large white peaches, peeled and halved

sea salt

1 small iceberg lettuce, shredded

125 g silken tofu

125 g chopped dates

125 g almonds, cut into halves lengthways

alfalfa sprouts, for garnishing

Rinse the peach halves in salted water to prevent browning and remove the stones. Place on a bed of lettuce on individual plates. Cream the tofu and put a spoonful in the centre of each peach. Arrange the dates and almonds on top with a few shreds of lettuce and garnish with a sprinkling of alfalfa sprouts.

the allergy exclusion diet

Spinach and tofu puffs

Good for: Rotation Diet, Day 3

Serves 4

FOR THE CHOUX PASTRY

4 tbsp sunflower seed oil or safflower oil

½ tsp sea salt

125 ml water

125 g rice flour

2 eggs

FOR THE FILLING

275 g spinach

275 g silken tofu

2 tsp umeboshi purée or pinch of nutmeg and sea salt

Preheat the oven to 170°C/Gas mark 3.

For the choux pastry, place the oil, salt and water in a pan and bring to the boil. Add the rice flour, beating with a wooden spoon to form a smooth dough. Allow to cool slightly and gradually beat in the eggs to form a paste. Using two spoons or an icing bag with a 2-cm diameter nozzle, drop eight mounds of dough on a baking sheet leaving room for the dough to expand. Bake for 20 to 25 minutes until they are firm and golden. Using a serrated knife, slice the top off each puff and leave to cool.

For the filling, wash and drain the spinach and cook it in its own juices for 2 to 3 minutes until tender. Drain thoroughly and chop. Mix with the silken tofu and flavourings and beat to form a smooth paste. Spoon the mixture into the choux puffs and replace the tops. Serve hot or cold.

This recipe may also be made up as a choux ring. Pipe the pastry on to the baking tray to form a 20-cm diameter ring leaving 10 cm clear in the centre.

Pears with stilton

Good for: Rotation Diet, Day 4

Serves 4

125 g crème fraîche
4 tbsp milk
50 g Stilton cheese
1 tsp poppy seeds
2 large pears

Place the crème fraîche and milk in a saucepan over a gentle heat. Crumble in the Stilton and stir until melted. Remove from the heat and mix in the poppy seeds and divide between four small serving plates.

Cut the pears in half lengthways and remove the cores. Cut each half into about eight segments, keeping the stalk end intact if possible and dip in and out of salt water to prevent browning. Arrange in a fan shape on top of the cheese sauce.

Open sandwiches

Good for: Elimination Diet, Day 18

Spread slices of rye/pumpernickel rye bread with tahini, hummus or nut spread and then add any of the following:

Fish salad: 1 sardine, 2 tomato wedges, lettuce leaf, cress and lemon slice.

Grape and tofu: slices of tofu, lettuce, tomato wedge and 1 or 2 black grapes, halved and deseeded.

Sprouted bean salad: alfalfa sprouts, cucumber slices and tomato wedge.

Game bird: breast of pheasant, watercress and slice of fresh orange.

Egg and tomato: slices of hard-boiled quail's eggs, 3 slices tomato, lettuce and parsley.

Prawn and salad: 50 g prawns, lettuce, 2 tomato wedges, lemon wedge and parsley.

Crab meal and salad: 50 g crab meat, lettuce, 2 walnut halves, cress and black olive.

Tuna fish roll

Good for: Rotation Diet, Day 4

Serves 4

450 g cooked sweet potato (pink fleshed if possible)

50 g tapioca flour

50 g butter (optional)

225 g cooked tuna fish, flaked

50 g crème fraîche or sheep's milk yoghurt

1 tbsp capers, chopped

25g horseradish, grated

1 tsp lemongrass

sea salt

watercress or mustard and cress, for garnishing

Preheat the oven to 160°C/Gas mark 3.

Mash the sweet potato, tapioca flour and butter, if using, until smooth. Take a Swiss roll tin, measuring approximately 30 x 23 cm and lined with greaseproof paper, and spread out the mixture 12-mm thick. Bake in the oven for 20 minutes.

Mix the tuna fish with the remaining ingredients and spread over the potato mixture. Hold one end of the greaseproof paper and roll up to make a roll. Leave to cool and cut into slices with a sharp knife. Serve on individual plates with a garnishing of watercress or mustard and cress salad.

POULTRY AND MEAT

Roast chicken with plum stuffing

Good for: Rotation Diet, Day 3

Serves 4

FOR THE STUFFING

125 g rice flakes

250 ml water

125 g sunflower seeds

4 red plums, stoned and chopped

sea salt

1 egg, beaten or 1 tsp sago flour

1.6 kg free-range chicken

8 plums

Preheat the oven to 190°C/Gas mark 5.

For the stuffing, soak the rice flakes in the water for 10 minutes. Mix the ingredients together and bind with the beaten egg or sago flour. Stuff into the neck end of the chicken. Place the chicken in a roasting tin and roast for 20 minutes. Reduce the oven temperature to 160°C/Gas mark 3 and continue roasting for a further hour until the chicken is golden brown and tender.

Remove the chicken from the oven 15 minutes before the end of the cooking time. Strain off any excess fat and place the plums around the chicken for the remaining cooking time. Transfer the chicken to a serving dish and surround with the plums. A purée of plums may be served as an accompaniment.

Curried chicken

Good for: Elimination Diet, Day 23

Serves 4

4 tbsp olive oil

675 g chicken fillet pieces

275 g onions

1 tbsp curry leaves, crushed

1 tsp ground coriander

1 tsp ground cumin

1 tsp turmeric

125 g creamed coconut

2 cloves garlic, crushed

1 tsp fresh ginger, mashed

sea salt

500 ml chicken stock or water

1 large unripe banana

Warm the olive oil and a little water in a heavy-based saucepan and seal the chicken pieces on both sides. Take out and place on a plate.

Gently cool fry the onions in the oil and water until transparent. Sprinkle in the spices, add the creamed coconut, garlic, ginger and salt. Return the chicken pieces, add the stock/water and finally the banana, cut into slices. Cover with a lid and simmer for 35 minutes, turning the chicken occasionally. Serve with rice, sliced tomatoes or pineapple pieces and chappatis (see page 212).

Chicken with beetroot

Good for: Rotation Diet, Day 3

Serves 4

4 chicken breasts

125 ml stock or water

pinch of nutmeg

sea salt

675 g beetroot, cooked and puréed

Place the chicken breasts in a saucepan and cook with the stock/water and seasoning until tender. Serve hot on a bed of puréed beetroot.

Turkey and mushroom fricassée

Good for: Elimination Diet, Day 15

Serves 4

600 ml game or vegetable stock

450 g turkey fillet

225 g mushrooms, sliced

2 sticks celery, sliced

1 onion, chopped

½ tsp ground mustard

2 cloves

sea salt

1 tbsp corn, barley or rice flour

Bring the stock to the boil and add the turkey, cut into strips, vegetables and seasoning. Cook gently for 10 to 15 minutes. Mix the flour with a little cold water and add to the pan to thicken the sauce.

Turkey and apricot pilaff

Good for: Elimination Diet, Day 8; Rotation Diet, Day 3

Serves 4

675 g turkey fillet

250 ml stock or water

sea salt

½ tsp nutmeg

125 g dried un-sulphured apricots, pre-soaked

50 g sultanas

225 g wholemeal basmati rice

Divide the turkey fillets into smaller pieces as required. Place in a saucepan and cover with stock/water (you may use the soaking water from the apricots). Add the salt, nutmeg and fruit and cook for 20 minutes until the chicken is cooked through.

Meanwhile, cook the rice in 500 ml salted water for about 15 minutes until almost tender. Mix with the turkey and fruit and cook for a further 10 minutes until the rice is tender and has absorbed some of the juices.

Stir-fry duck with mangetout

Good for: Rotation Diet, Day 3

Serves 4

450 g duckling breasts, cut into thin strips

225 g mangetout, topped and tailed

125 g bean sprouts

2 heads chicory, sliced

2 tsps honey

1 tbsp Tamari soya sauce

50 g almonds, cut lengthways, for garnishing

Heat a little water in a wok and add the strips of duck. Cook for 5 minutes and then add the mangetout, bean sprouts and chicory. Cook for a further 7 to 10 minutes. Stir in the honey and soya sauce and garnish with almonds. Serve with brown rice.

Wild duck with pineapple

Good for: Preliminary Diet; Elimination Diet, Day 27

Serves 4

900 g oven-ready wild duck
1 carrot, cut into strips
1 celery stalk, sliced
250 ml stock or mineral water
1 bay leaf
1 sprig thyme
sea salt
1 small pineapple

Preheat the oven to 190°C/Gas mark 5.

Place the duck in an ovenproof casserole dish and add the vegetables, stock/water, bay leaf, thyme and salt and cook for 1½ hours, reducing the oven temperature to 160°C/Gas mark 3 after the first 15 minutes. Baste from time to time and add more water if necessary. When cooked, lift onto a serving dish.

Prepare the pineapple by removing the skin and cutting into slices 1-cm thick and cook in the remaining juice, simmering for approximately 2 minutes. Remove the bay leaf and thyme. Garnish the duck with pineapple and pour over the juice.

Roast duck with orange and grapefruit sauce

Good for: Preliminary Diet; Elimination Diet, Day 19

Serves 4

1.8 kg oven-ready duck

2 small grapefruit

2 bay leaves

3 oranges

1 tsp cornflour or tapioca flour

2 tbsp honey

Preheat the oven to 190°C/Gas mark 5.

Prick the duck all over with a fork. Sprinkle with salt and place half a grapefruit and 2 bay leaves in the body cavity.

Place on a rack or trivet, breast side down, in a roasting pan and roast in the oven for 30 minutes. Reduce the oven temperature to 160°C/Gas mark 3 and cook for a further 1½ hours. Baste from time to time and you can also, if you wish, remove the pan from the oven and pour off the excess fat and use this for roasting potatoes.

To prepare the sauce, squeeze the juice from the remaining grapefruit half and the juice from 1 orange. Peel the other grapefruit and 2 oranges and cut the peel into thin strips. Bring some water to the boil and blanche the strips of peel for 2 to 3 minutes, drain and put to one side. Cut the oranges into thin slices and divide the grapefruit into segments.

When the duck is cooked, pour off the cooking juices and place the duck on a serving dish and keep warm in the turned off oven. Skim off the excess fat from the roasting pan and place over a medium heat. Mix the cornflour to a smooth paste with a little cold water and add to the juices in the pan. Add the orange and grapefruit juices, the strips of peel and the honey and simmer, stirring for 2 to 3 minutes until the sauce thickens. Pour around the duck. Garnish with the orange slices arranged along the breast and the grapefruit segments round the dish and serve immediately.

Game bird casserole

Good for: Preliminary Diet; Elimination Diet, Day 7

Serves 4

A brace of grouse, partridge or 3 pigeons

3 to 4 carrots

1 parsnip

2 sticks of celery, sliced

2 tsp chopped parsley

sea salt

600 ml boiling mineral water

2 tsp tapioca flour

Preheat the oven to 190°C/Gas mark 5.

Place the game birds in an ovenproof casserole dish. Add the vegetables, left whole or cut where necessary, parsley and salt and pour in the boiling water. Cook for 1½ hours reducing the temperature of the oven to 160°C/Gas mark 3 after the first 20 minutes.

Place the game birds and the vegetables on a hot serving dish. Skim off any fat and use the cooking juices to make a gravy, using a little tapioca flour mixed with some cold water, to thicken.

Roast quails with spring onion rice and cranberry sauce

Good for: Elimination Diet, Day 11

Serves 4

6 to 8 oven-ready quails (allow 1 to 2 per person)

sea salt

FOR THE SPRING ONION RICE

125 g spring onions

300 g long grain rice (a little wild rice may be used)

2 bay leaves

850 ml water

FOR THE SAUCE

225 g cranberries

125 ml water

1 clove garlic (optional)

grated zest and juice of 1 orange (optional)

pinch of cinnamon

2 tbsp maple syrup or to taste

Preheat the oven to 180°C/Gas mark 4.

Place the quails in a casserole dish and sprinkle with salt. Cover and cook for 30 minutes.

To cook the rice, cut the spring onions into 2-cm lengths and add the rice, bay leaves, salt and water. Bring to the boil, cover and simmer for 20 to 25 minutes until cooked. Remove the bay leaves before serving.

To make the cranberry sauce, place all the ingredients in a pan except for the maple syrup and simmer gently for 2 to 3 minutes until the cranberries are tender. Add fruit sugar to taste.

Place the rice on a serving dish and arrange the quails on the top and serve with cranberry sauce.

Pigeon with prunes

Good for: Rotation Diet, Day 3

Serves 4

8 pigeon breasts

600 ml stock or water

225 g cooked prunes

2 tsp fresh tarragon chopped

pinch of nutmeg

sea salt

2 tsp sago flour

Place the pigeon breasts in a flameproof casserole dish and add the stock/water mixed with a little prune juice, and the remaining ingredients, except for the sago flour. Cover with a lid and cook over a gentle heat for 20 minutes. Lift out the pigeon breasts and place on a serving dish.

Mix the sago flour with some cold water and stir into the cooking stock to make a sauce. Pour over the pigeon breasts and arrange the prunes around. Serve on a bed of rice with diced French beans and peas.

Pot roast pheasant/wild game bird

Good for: Rotation Diet, Day 3

Serves 4

1 pheasant

salt

nutmeg

This is an excellent way of cooking game birds when the age and tenderness of the meat is unknown. Some pheasants are fed on corn and this may affect some people. The same goes for corn-fed poultry.

Preheat the oven to 190°C/Gas mark 5.

Place the pheasant in a heavy-based casserole dish. Add enough boiling water to half cover and season with salt and nutmeg. Cover and cook for 1 to 1½ hours, reducing the temperature to 160°C/Gas mark 3 after the first 15 minutes, until the meat is tender and is just beginning to fall away from the bone.

Rabbit/hare hot pot

Good for: Preliminary Diet; Rotation Diet, Day 1

Serves 4

900 g rabbit/hare portions

1 parsnip, diced

4 carrots, sliced

3 sticks celery, sliced

125 g pot barley (use rice for Preliminary Diet)

sea salt or kelp

1 litre boiling water

2 tbsp freshly chopped parsley, for garnishing

Arrange the rabbit or hare portions in a heavy-based saucepan. Add the vegetables, barley and salt and pour over the boiling water. Bring to the boil and simmer gently for 1½ hours. Add the chopped parsley and serve.

Pot roast rabbit with mushroom and fennel stuffing

Good for: Rotation Diet, Day 1

Serves 4

FOR THE STUFFING

125 g breadcrumbs or millet flakes

125 g mushrooms, chopped

grated zest and juice of 1 lemon

1 bulb fennel, chopped

3 tbsp fresh parsley, chopped

1 tsp chopped chervil, if available

sea salt

1 large rabbit, skinned

600 ml stock or water

Preheat the oven to 180°C/Gas mark 4.

Mix together the ingredients for the stuffing adding a little water if necessary. Stuff the body of the rabbit and bring the open sides together, securing with string or skewers. Place in a casserole dish, pour over the stock/water and place the lid on the top. Cook in the oven for 15 minutes. Reduce the temperature to 160°C/Gas mark 3 and cook for a further 45 minutes. Allow the rabbit to rest for 10 minutes before carving.

Lamb noisettes

Good for: Elimination Diet, Day 28

Serves 4

FOR THE TOPPING

50 g rice flakes

1 large onion, chopped

sea salt

knob of butter

125 ml stock

1 egg yolk

1 tbsp yoghurt

8 lamb cutlets trimmed

grated cheese

FOR GARNISHING

125 g mushrooms, chopped

knob of butter

sea salt

1 tbsp mixed herbs, e.g. tarragon, mint, parsley

Preheat the oven to 160°C/Gas mark 3.

To prepare the topping, place the rice, onion, salt and a knob of butter in a pan and pour over the stock. Bring to the boil and simmer for 35 minutes. Sieve the rice mixture and add the egg yolk and yoghurt to make a smooth purée.

Prepare the cutlets, grill on one side only for about 5 minutes with the bones all running the same way. Cover the cooked side of each cutlet with the purée, shaping it on neatly. Sprinkle with grated cheese and arrange on a baking tray and cook in the oven for 20 minutes.

For the garnish, peel and trim the mushrooms. Chop the stalks and cool fry in butter for about 1 minute, without allowing the butter to brown. Add seasoning and herbs. Fill into the hollow of the mushrooms and pour over a little melted butter. Put on to a tray and cook in the oven for with the cutlets for 10 minutes.

Lamb burgers

Good for: Preliminary Diet; Rotation Diet, Day 4

Serves 4

175 g lean lamb
50 g lamb's liver
125 g chestnut flour
sea salt

Mince the lamb and the liver. Mix together with the chestnut flour and seasoning and shape into 4 burgers about 2.5 cm thick, or use a burger press. Grill for 4 to 5 minutes on each side.

Vegetarian/lamb shepherd's pie

Good for: Elimination Diet, Day 28

Serves 4

2 onions, sliced
2 carrots, diced
1 stick celery, diced
1 courgette, diced
225 g brown lentils, sprouted and cooked
125 g buckwheat or pot barley, cooked
125 g hazelnuts, chopped
tamari or teriyaki soya sauce
450 g potatoes, cooked and mashed
50 g Cheddar cheese (optional)
NB: Lentils, buckwheat and hazelnuts may be replaced with 450 g of cooked, minced lamb.

Preheat the oven to 160°C/Gas mark 3.

Steam or boil the vegetables until tender. Mix with the lentils, buckwheat, hazelnuts and soya sauce and turn into a well-oiled ovenproof dish. Top with the mashed potato, sprinkle with cheese, if using, and bake for 30 to 35 minutes.

Pot roast leg of lamb

Good for: Elimination Diet, Day 26

Serves 4

1.8 kg leg of lamb
sea salt
3 to 4 sprigs of rosemary
2 carrots, sliced
1 parsnip, sliced lengthways
2 sticks of celery, sliced
1 leek, sliced (optional)
1 tsp tomato purée (optional)
500 ml stock or water

Preheat oven to 180°C/Gas mark 4.

Trim off excess fat from the lamb, season with salt and lay in the sprigs of rosemary over the joint. Place in a roasting pan and put in the oven for 15 minutes to seal. Remove from the oven and transfer to a large casserole dish. Add the vegetables, tomato purée and stock/water and cover with the lid. Return to the oven, reducing the temperature to 150°C/Gas mark 2 and cook for a further 2 hours, until very tender.

Place the lamb on a serving dish with the vegetables and keep warm. Strain off the juices, skimming off any excess fat and serve in a jug. This can be thickened with sago, tapioca or any permissible flour.

Shoulder of lamb with apricot, raisin and oat stuffing

Good for: Elimination Diet, Day 16

Serves 4

FOR THE STUFFING

225 g fresh apricots, chopped

50 g raisins

50 g oat flakes

2 tsp fresh tarragon, parsley or chosen herb

sea salt

1 tsp tapioca flour

250 ml stock or water

1 boned shoulder of lamb

Preheat the oven to 180°C/Gas mark 4 and reduce to 160°C/Gas mark 3 after the first 15 minutes.

For the stuffing, put the apricots, raisins, oats and seasoning in a bowl and bind together with the tapioca and stock/water. Place the stuffing into the cavity of the meat and tie with string or secure with skewers. Roast for 1½ to 2 hours and serve with gravy.

Creamy lamb with rye spaghetti

Good for: Elimination Diet, Day 20

Serves 4

250 ml lamb stock

450 g lean lamb, cut into strips

1 large red pepper, deseeded and cut into 5-cm strips

225 g courgette, cut into 5-cm strips

1 clove garlic

½ tsp ground rosemary

pinch of nutmeg

sea salt

1 tbsp sago/tapioca/cornflour (optional)

275 g sheep's milk yoghurt

275 g rye spaghetti, barley or buckwheat pasta, cooked

Pour the stock into a saucepan and bring to the boil. Add the lamb, vegetables and seasoning and cook gently for 15 minutes. Thicken with the sago flour/tapioca/cornflour if necessary. Just before serving, stir in the yoghurt and serve with rye pasta.

Devilled lamb's kidneys

Good for: Preliminary Diet

Serves 4

4 lamb's kidneys

2 tbsp gram flour (chickpea flour)

sea salt (optional)

250 ml lamb stock

Wash the kidneys in cold water. Dry and remove the cores. Cut into thin slices and roll each slice in the gram flour, sprinkled with a little salt if liked. Heat the stock in a pan, add the kidneys and cook gently for 4 to 5 minutes

Moussaka

Good for: Elimination Diet, Day 24

Serves 4

4 large aubergines, sliced

sea salt

2 large onions, chopped

1 clove garlic, crushed

2 tbsp sesame seed oil

450 g lean minced lamb or 225 g aduki beans, sprouted and cooked

225 g tomatoes, skinned and chopped

1 green pepper, deseeded and chopped

1 tbsp tomato purée

½ tsp oregano

sea salt or kelp

FOR THE SAUCE

2 free-range eggs or soya egg replacer

250 ml goat's milk yoghurt

½ tsp allspice or nutmeg

½ tsp ground mustard

½ salt to taste

50 g hard goat's cheese, grated

Preheat the oven to 160°C/Gas mark 3.

Sprinkle the aubergine slices with salt to remove bitterness. Leave for 30 minutes, drain and dry on kitchen paper. Steam or boil in a little water until tender and set to one side.

Cool fry the onions and garlic in oil and water until transparent. Add the lamb/aduki beans, tomatoes, pepper and flavourings and cook for 10 minutes. Using a well-oiled shallow ovenproof baking dish, arrange the aubergine slices and the lamb/aduki bean mixture in layers.

For the sauce, beat together the eggs and yoghurt and add the spices and seasoning. Pour over the top and sprinkle with grated cheese. Bake for 30 to 40 minutes.

Braised venison with juniper

Good for: Preliminary Diet; Elimination Diet, Day 10

Serves 4

4 venison steaks
2 sticks celery, sliced
2 carrots, diced
8 juniper berries
sea salt
500 ml stock or mineral water
1 tbsp sago or tapioca flour
chopped parsley, for garnishing

Preheat the oven to 160°C/Gas mark 3.

Grill the steaks on both sides, to seal. Place in an ovenproof casserole dish. Add the vegetables, juniper berries and salt and pour over the stock/water. Cook for 1 hour until the meat is tender. Mix the sago/tapioca flour with a little cold water and add to the juices to thicken the sauce. Garnish with chopped parsley and serve with red currant sauce (see page 196).

Venison steak burgers

Good for: Elimination Diet, Day 17

Serves 4

450 g minced venison
50 g fine oatmeal or gram flour
125 g chestnut flour
1 tsp ground coriander
1 tsp chopped chives
sea salt

Mix together all the ingredients. Shape into four burgers about 2-cm thick. Grill for 5 to 7 minutes on each side.

Venison and cucumber stir-fry

Good for: Rotation Diet, Day 2

Serves 4

450 g lean venison cut into thin strips
2 cloves garlic
1 tsp grated ginger
225 g baby sweetcorn
1 red pepper, deseeded and cut into strips
½ cucumber, halved lengthways and sliced
sea salt

Heat a little water in a large frying pan or wok. Add the venison and cook for 5 minutes. Add the rest of the ingredients in order of cooking time, leaving the cucumber until the end. Season to taste.

Fillet of beef with caper sauce

Good for: Rotation Diet, Day 4

Serves 4

FOR THE CAPER SAUCE

3 tbsp capers
75 g anchovy fillets (in brine)
1 tsp ground lemongrass
1 cup sour cream
sea salt

4 fillets of steak from organically reared beef
sea salt

For the sauce, place all the ingredients in a liquidiser and blend to a smooth sauce.

Preheat the grill. Sprinkle the steaks with salt and grill for 3 to 5 minutes on each side according to preference. Spoon the sauce on top and serve immediately.

Pot roast brisket of beef with horseradish sauce

Good for: Rotation Diet, Day 4

Serves 4

1 to 1.5 kg brisket or silverside joint of organically reared beef

1 litre stock or water

450 g diced vegetables, e.g. swede, turnip, kohlrabi

1 tsp mustard seeds

sea salt

tapioca flour

Preheat the oven to 190°C/Gas mark 5.

Put the joint of beef in an open ovenproof casserole dish. Place in the oven for 20 minutes to seal. Remove the meat from the oven and add the stock/water, vegetables and seasoning. Reduce the oven temperature to 150°C/Gas mark 2, place the lid on the top of the casserole dish and cook for 2½ hours.

Place the meat on a serving dish and strain off the juices and use some to make a gravy – skim off any fat, reheat and stir in some tapioca flour, mixed with a little cold water. Keep stirring until the gravy thickens.

Beef stew with barley dumplings

Good for: Elimination Diet, Day 12

Serves 4

600 ml stock or water

450 g organically reared beef steak, cubed

2 carrots, diced

1 parsnip, diced

2 sticks celery, sliced

2 sprigs fresh thyme or ½ tsp dried

sea salt

FOR THE BARLEY DUMPLINGS
(see page 193)

Preheat the oven to 150°C/Gas mark 2.

Bring the stock/water to boiling point in an ovenproof casserole dish and add the beef, vegetables and seasoning and return to boiling point. Add the barley dumplings and place the casserole in the oven and cook for 1½ hours until the meat is tender.

Chilli con carne

Good for: Elimination Diet, Day 24

Serves 4

500 ml stock

450 g organic lean beef steak, cut into cubes

2 onions, chopped

2 cloves garlic, crushed

½ tsp cayenne pepper

1 tsp oregano

sea salt

6 tomatoes, skinned and chopped

175 g red kidney beans, sprouted and cooked

1 tbsp barley or rice flour

Pour the stock into a heavy-based saucepan and bring to the boil. Add all the ingredients except the tomatoes and kidney beans. Cover and cook for 1 hour or until the meat is tender.

Add the tomatoes and kidney beans and cook for a further 15 minutes. Mix the barley flour with a little cold water and stir into the juices to thicken.

Pork, apple and chestnut pie

Good for: Elimination Diet, Day 13

Serves 4

FOR THE FILLING

225 g minced pork

225 g chestnuts, cooked and broken into pieces

225 g cox's apples, peeled and sliced

4 quail's eggs or 2 tbsp soya egg replacer, beaten

125 ml stock

1 tsp fresh thyme or ½ tsp dried

sea salt

FOR THE SWEET POTATO AND BUCKWHEAT PASTRY

125 g sweet potato, baked and mashed

50 g buckwheat flour

50 g soya flour

125 ml olive oil

1 tsp baking powder (wheat free)

sea salt

water to mix

1 egg, beaten

Preheat the oven to 160°C/Gas mark 3 and line and grease a 20-cm flan case.

For the filling, mix together all the ingredients.

For the pastry, mix the ingredients and form into a firm dough. Roll out two-thirds of the pastry and line the base of the flan case. Prick the base and spread with the filling. Cover with the remaining pastry and seal the edges. Brush with a little beaten egg and pierce the lid of the pie to allow steam to escape. Bake for 50 minutes and serve hot or cold.

Pork tenderloin with prune, anchovy and almond stuffing

Good for: Elimination Diet, Day 21

Serves 4

18 large prunes

8 anchovy fillets

8 blanched almonds

2 outdoor reared/organic pork tenderloins

600 ml vegetable or marrow bone stock

1 tbsp arrowroot

salt

Soak the prunes overnight and stone before using.

Preheat the oven to 180°C/Gas mark 4.

To stuff eight prunes, wrap an anchovy fillet round a blanched almond and fill the cavity of the prune.

To prepare the tenderloins, slit down one long side, just over half-way through, and open out. Lay the stuffed prunes on one opened out tenderloin. Lay the second tenderloin on top and tie together at intervals with string. Place in an ovenproof casserole and bake for 40 minutes, reducing the oven temperature to 160°C/Gas mark 3 after the first 20 minutes.

Cook the remaining prunes for 1 to 2 minutes. Drain and place on one side, keeping the liquid to add to the sauce.

Remove the pork tenderloin from the casserole, carve into slices and arrange on a hot serving dish. Use the cooking juices, stock, seasoning and the prune juice to make a sauce, and thicken with arrowroot. Pour over the meat and garnish with the remaining prunes.

Sweet and sour vegetables/pork

Good for: Elimination Diet, Day 21

Serves 4

FOR THE SWEET AND SOUR SAUCE

125 ml water

2 tsp cornflour/tapioca/sago

2 tbsp soya sauce

2 tbsp wine vinegar

1 tbsp clear honey

1 tbsp tomato purée

450 g lean organic pork, cut into strips (optional)

225 g courgettes, sliced

225 g water chestnuts

125 g baby sweetcorn

125 g sugar peas

1 carrot, cut into julienne strips

1 red/green pepper, deseeded and sliced

½ cucumber, diced

2 tbsp sesame seed oil

To make the sweet and sour sauce, cream together the cornflour and water, mix in the remaining ingredients and pour into a saucepan. Gently cook, stirring all the time, until the sauce thickens.

For the pork and vegetables, heat some water in the bottom of the wok and cook the pork. Add the vegetables in order of cooking time until just tender. Add the sweet and sour sauce, tossing the vegetables until all are coated and the sauce thickens. Just before serving, stir in the sesame seed oil.

Pork and pineapple kebabs

Good for: Rotation Diet, Day 2

Serves 4

675 g lean organic pork, cut into 2.5-cm cubes

1 pineapple, skinned and cut into cubes

2 green peppers, deseeded and cut into 2-cm pieces

8 bay leaves

2 tsp freshly chopped thyme

sea salt

Thread the pork, pineapple cubes, green pepper pieces and bay leaves on to four long skewers. Sprinkle with thyme and salt and place the kebabs on an oiled grill rack. Grill under a medium heat for 10 to 15 minutes, turning frequently.

Pig's liver and onions

Good for: Rotation Diet, Day 2

Serves 4

2 tbsp olive oil

3 onions, sliced

450 g organic pig's liver, thinly sliced

1 tbsp fine oatmeal

sea salt

250 ml pork or vegetable stock or water

1 tsp cornflour

Warm the oil with a little water in a heavy-based frying pan. Cool fry the onions until transparent and place on a serving dish and keep warm.

Roll the slices of liver in the oatmeal seasoned with salt, and gently cool fry on both sides until just cooked (2 to 3 minutes). Place on top of the onions.

To make a gravy, add the stock to the pan, adding a little cornflour mixed with cold water if necessary.

Meatballs in tomato sauce

Good for: Rotation Diet, Day 2

Serves 4

FOR THE SAUCE

6 fresh tomatoes, skinned and chopped

1 pepper, deseeded and diced

2 spring onions, chopped

1 clove garlic, crushed

1 tsp basil

½ tsp cayenne pepper

sea salt

450 ml stock or water

FOR THE MEATBALLS

450 g minced meat (pork or venison)

1 large onion, chopped (not fried)

2 cloves garlic, crushed

2 tbsp tomato purée

2 tbsp fine oatmeal or maize meal

1 tsp ginger grated

½ tsp ground cardamom

½ tsp chilli powder (optional)

sea salt

For the sauce, cook the vegetables in the stock/water for 15 minutes until tender.

For the meatballs, mix together all the ingredients either by hand or in a food mixer and mould into approximately eight meatballs. Bring the stock to the boil and add the meatballs. Pour over the tomato sauce and simmer gently for 30 minutes.

Roast pork/wild boar with juniper

Good for: Rotation Diet, Day 2

Serves 4

1 tbsp fine oatmeal

2 tbsp freshly chopped sage

10 juniper berries, crushed

2 cloves garlic, crushed

sea salt

1 kg boned loin of organically reared pork

Preheat the oven to 180°C/Gas mark 4.

Mix together the oatmeal, sage, juniper berries, garlic and seasoning. Trim off the skin and excess fat from the pork and cut some deep slashes in the top and sides. Place in a roasting tray and press in the herb and juniper mixture. Roast for approximately 1 hour until thoroughly cooked.

Wild boar cutlets with mushroom sauce

Good for: Elimination Diet, Day 13

Serves 4

4 to 6 wild boar loan cutlets, trimmed

600 ml stock

225 g small turnips, diced

1 tsp ground mustard seeds

sea salt

125 g button mushrooms

sago or tapioca flour

Grill the cutlets on both sides to seal the juices. Place in a pan with the stock, turnips and seasoning and bring to the boil. Cover and simmer for 30 minutes and then add the mushrooms. Cook for a further 5 minutes. Thicken the juices with a little sago or tapioca flour.

Fruit-roasted leg of wild boar

Good for: Elimination Diet, Day 25

Serves 8 to 10

FOR THE FRUIT COATING

175 g dried apricots, finely chopped

175 g dried prunes, finely chopped

10 juniper berries, crushed

grated zest and juice of 1 orange

2 tbsp oatmeal

1 tsp allspice

sea salt

1.6 to 2 kg whole leg of wild boar

600 ml prune juice

arrowroot (optional)

Preheat the oven to 180°C/Gas mark 4 and reduce to 160°C/Gas mark 3 after the first 20 minutes.

Mix together the ingredients for the fruit coating using a little of the prune juice to bind if necessary.

Trim off the skin and any excess fat from the leg and place, inner side down, in a well-oiled roasting pan. Coat the upper surface with the fruit mixture, pressing it down evenly as you go. Pour the prune juice around the joint and cook for 40 minutes per 450 g weight, basting with the prune juice from time to time, until thoroughly cooked.

Transfer to a warm serving dish. Add some water to the roasting pan and boil up the juices. Skim off any fat, thicken with arrowroot or similar flour if you wish, and serve with the meat.

FISH

Red mullet with seasoned rice stuffing

Good for: Preliminary Diet

Serves 4

4 red mullet, about 175 g each, cleaned and scaled

sea salt

FOR THE STUFFING

175 g long grain rice, cooked

50 g pine nuts

50 g sultanas

50 g chopped olives (not in vinegar)

1 tsp ground lemongrass

1 tsp coriander leaves

sea salt

Preheat the oven to 180°C/Gas mark 4.

Mix together the ingredients for the stuffing and fill the cavity of each fish and secure with a skewer.

Place the fish in a well-oiled baking tray, sprinkle with salt and bake for 30 to 35 minutes.

Rolled plaice with spinach

Good for: Elimination Diet, Day 10

Serves 4

675 g spinach

4 fillets of plaice

50 g maize or millet flour

50 g ground cashew nuts

sea salt

sprigs of parsley, for garnishing

Preheat the oven to 160°C/Gas mark 3.

Thoroughly wash and steam the spinach in its own moisture, until tender. Mash with a fork and place in a well-oiled casserole dish.

Cut the plaice fillets in two lengthways and roll up each half, securing with a cocktail stick. Arrange on top of the spinach and sprinkle with a mixture of millet flour, ground cashew nuts and sea salt. Cover and cook for 30 minutes. Serve garnished with parsley.

Fisherman's pie

Good for: Rotation Diet, Day 4

Serves 4

450 g fillet of cod or similar fish

250 ml sheep's or goat's milk

sea salt

1 tbsp tapioca flour

450 g yam, cooked and mashed

Preheat the oven to 160°C/Gas mark 3.

Place the fish in a pan and cover with the milk and a pinch of salt. Bring to the boil and simmer very gently for 4 to 5 minutes until just cooked. Strain off the milk and place the fish in a pie dish.

Mix the flour with a little water and add to the milk. Cook, stirring until the sauce thickens and pour over the fish. Top with mashed yam and bake for 30 minutes.

Buckwheat and walnut coated herrings

Good for: Rotation Diet, Day 4

Serves 4

4 herrings

FOR THE TOPPING

50 g buckwheat flakes

50 g walnuts, finely chopped

125 g sheep's yoghurt

1 tsp ground mustard seeds

25 g butter (optional)

sea salt or kelp

Wash and scale the herrings and cut off the heads. Slit the herrings open and remove the guts and backbones. Grill the herrings on both sides until almost cooked.

For the topping, mix together the ingredients and spread over the cutlets. Grill for a further minute.

Grilled halibut with anchovy butter

Good for: Rotation Diet, Day 4

Serves 4

4 halibut steaks

FOR THE ANCHOVY BUTTER

75 g anchovy fillets

125 g unsalted butter

Preheat and grease the grill pan and grill the halibut for 6 to 8 minutes until just cooked through. There should be no need to turn.

To prepare the butter, rinse and dry the anchovies. Chop finely and rub through a sieve. Beat into the butter and form into butter pats and serve with the halibut.

Fresh salmon with raspberry coulis

Good for: Elimination Diet, Day 14

Serves 4

4 wild salmon fillets

sea salt

225 g fresh raspberries

125 ml water

1 tbsp fruit sugar

Sprinkle the salmon fillets with salt and poach for 4 to 5 minutes.

Place the raspberries in a saucepan with the water and fruit sugar and bring to the boil. Simmer until the raspberries begin to break up. Liquidise, strain and serve with the salmon.

Salmon and tomato fish cakes

Good for: Elimination Diet, Day 26

Serves 4

225 g flaked cooked salmon

225 g cooked and mashed potato or yam

2 to 3 tomatoes, skinned and chopped

25 g capers, chopped

1 onion, finely chopped

1 tsp arrowroot or tapioca flour

1 tbsp lemon juice or 1 tsp lemongrass

1 tsp thyme

sea salt or kelp

2 tbsp maize or millet flour for coating

Preheat the oven to 160°C/Gas mark 3.

Mix all the ingredients together and mould into four fish cakes and roll in the maize flour. Bake for 25 minutes.

Prawn or tofu chow mein

Good for: Elimination Diet, Day 26

Serves 4

25 cm wakame seaweed
225 g vermicelli (rice noodles)
225 g bean sprouts
225 g water chestnuts, sliced
125 g organic mushrooms, sliced
2 carrots, thinly sliced diagonally
125 ml vegetable stock
350 g shelled prawns or 350 g tofu, cut into squares
1 tbsp tamari soya sauce
1 tbsp organic white wine (optional)
sesame seed oil, for garnishing

Wash and soak the wakame seaweed for 10 minutes. Drain and cut into 2 to 3-cm pieces. The soaking water may be used to cook the noodles. Bring the water to the boil and cook the vermicelli until just soft. Drain well and place on a serving dish and keep warm.

Heat some water in a wok or saucepan and cook the vegetables for 5 minutes. Add the stock and bring to the boil. Add the prawns, seaweed, soya sauce and wine and cook for another 3 minutes. Place on the serving dish in the centre of the noodles and sprinkle with sesame seed oil.

Grilled trout fillets with tropical fruit

Good for: Rotation Diet, Day 1

Serves 4

1 large mango

4 pieces of trout fillet (not farmed)

sea salt

1 tsp ground coriander

1 star fruit

2 tbsp fresh coriander leaves, chopped, for garnishing

To prepare the mango, hold upright and take a slice off each side, cutting down as near to the stone as possible, then cutting the smaller pieces off the ends. Skin and cut into matchstick pieces.

Place the trout in a grill pan, sprinkle with salt and ground coriander and grill for 5 to 7 minutes. Arrange on a bed of the mango and sliced star fruit and garnish with chopped coriander leaves.

the allergy exclusion diet

Stuffed squid

Good for: Rotation Diet, Day 1

Serves 4

1 kg small squid, cleaned and prepared

FOR THE STUFFING

50 g breadcrumbs or cooked millet

2 sticks celery, finely diced

2 tbsp fresh parsley, chopped

3 tbsp sesame seed oil

rind of 1 lemon

sea salt or kelp

3 carrots, cut into matchsticks

250 ml vegetable stock

chopped parsley, for garnishing

lemon wedges, for garnishing

Preheat the oven to 160°C/Gas mark 3.

Mix together the ingredients for the stuffing and stuff the squid bodies with the mixture. Sew up or fasten the opening with a cocktail stick. Place in an ovenproof dish, with the carrots and pour over the stock. Bake for 45 minutes and serve hot with a sprinkling of parsley and lemon wedges.

Seafood paella

Good for: Elimination Diet, Day 22

Serves 6 to 8

450 g fresh mussels
1 bay leaf
1 litre water or vegetable stock
2 tbsp olive oil
1 onion, peeled and chopped
2 cloves garlic
350 g long-grain rice
sea salt
1 tsp ground lemongrass
Saffron

225 g tomatoes, skinned and chopped
1 red pepper, deseeded and sliced
125 g peas
450 g small squid, cleaned, prepared and cut into rings
175 g prepared scallops

FOR THE GARNISHING
125 g black olives (preservative free)
1 lemon cut into wedges
2 tsp fresh coriander, chopped

Scrub the mussels, removing the thread-like beards and discarding any that do not close when tapped. Place in a pan with water and a bay leaf and cook for 5 minutes until the shells open. Strain off the liquid and make up to 1 litre with water or vegetable stock. Reserve 8 to 10 mussels in their shells and shell the rest, discarding any that have not opened.

Warm the oil and a little water in a large shallow saucepan or paella pan and cool fry the onion and garlic until soft. Stir in the rice and cook for 1 to 2 minutes. Add the stock, salt, lemongrass and saffron, bring to the boil and cook for 15 minutes. Stir in the tomatoes, red pepper, peas, squid, scallops and shelled mussels and cook for 4 to 5 minutes until the rice is tender. Serve garnished with mussels in their shells, black olives, wedges of lemon and a sprinkling of coriander leaves.

the allergy exclusion diet

VEGETARIAN

Spanish omelette
Good for: Elimination Diet, Day 27
Serves 4

2 tbsp olive oil
1 onion, chopped
2 cloves garlic, crushed
2 courgettes, thinly sliced
2 tomatoes skinned, deseeded and chopped
1 tsp oregano
sea salt
4 free-range chicken eggs

Warm the olive oil and a little water in a pan and cool fry the onions until soft. Add the garlic, courgette and tomatoes and seasoning, cover the pan and cook gently for 7 to 10 minutes.

Beat the eggs and stir into the vegetables. Cook over gently heat for 2 to 3 minutes until the underside is cooked. Place the pan under a preheated grill and cook the top of the omelette for another 2 to 3 minutes until set. Cut into quarters and serve.

Millet and cashew nut risotto
Good for: Elimination Diet, Day 10
Serves 4
2 sticks celery, sliced
225 g millet, cooked
125 g cashew nuts
50 g black olives (preservative free)

Blanche the sliced celery by immersing in boiling water for 30 seconds. Mix the ingredients together and serve hot or cold.

Millet, lentil and brazil nut loaf

Good for: Preliminary Diet; Elimination Diet, Day 26

Serves 4

125 g millet

125 g green lentils, sprouted

250 ml vegetable stock or mineral water

1 tbsp tapioca flour

125 g Brazil nuts, roughly chopped

2 sticks celery, diced

1 tbsp sage

sea salt

Preheat the oven to 160°C/Gas mark 3.

Cook the millet and lentils in the stock/water for 15 minutes and mix with the rest of the ingredients in a food mixer or with a wooden spoon. Oil a loaf tin or deep pie dish and press the mixture well in. Bake for 45 minutes or until the top of the loaf is brown and firm to the touch. Serve hot or cold.

Barley, cashew and vegetable loaf

Good for: Preliminary Diet; Elimination Diet, Day 25; Rotation Diet, Day 1

Serves 4

225 g pot barley, cooked

125 g shiitake mushrooms, diced

125 g cashew nuts, chopped

2 carrots, grated

2 tbsp barley flour

2 tbsp freshly chopped coriander leaves

125 ml stock or water

sea salt or 1 tsp barley miso

Preheat the oven to 160°C/Gas mark 3.

Mix together all the ingredients and turn into a lined loaf tin. Bake for about 50 minutes until firm.

Sweet potato and seafood bakes

Good for: Preliminary Diet; Elimination Diet, Day 6

Serves 4

225 g sweet potato
225 g tuna fish, cooked
basil
sea salt
quinoa flour

Preheat the oven to 160°C/Gas mark 3.

Cook the sweet potatoes by boiling or baking. Do not fry. A large sweet potato weighing 450 g will take 1 hour to cook at 160°C/Gas mark 3.

Mix together the sweet potato and tuna fish. Add the basil and salt. Make into cakes and roll each one in the quinoa flour. Bake for 20 minutes, turning once.

For larger quantities, the mixture may be formed into a roll on a lightly floured board and cut into slices before shaping and flouring. Useful for freezing.

Courgette bakes may be made in a similar way, substituting grated courgette for tuna fish.

Aduki bean burgers

Good for: Rotation Diet, Day 3

Serves 4

225 g sprouted and cooked aduki beans
225 g cooked organic short grain rice
125 g ground almonds
1 tbsp sago flour
1 tsp freshly chopped tarragon
sea salt

Mash together all the ingredients and shape into burgers or use a burger press. Grill for 4 to 5 minutes on each side under low to moderate heat.

Brazil nut bean burgers

Good for: Elimination Diet, Day 9

Serves 4

225 g black-eyed beans, sprouted and cooked

125 g Brazil nuts, soaked and chopped

125 g buckwheat flakes

2 tbsp safflower oil

1 tsp dried sage

sea salt

1 tsp millet flour

Preheat the oven to 160°C/Gas mark 3.

Mix together all the ingredients, adding a little water if necessary, and mould into burgers or use a burger press. Roll in millet flour and bake for 20 minutes.

Brazil nut roast

Good for: Rotation Diet, Day 2

Serves 4

175 g maize flour

50 g oatflakes

175 g Brazil nuts, chopped

175 g courgette, grated

2 onions, finely chopped

250 ml water

1 tbsp freshly chopped sage

sea salt

1 tbsp olive oil

Preheat the oven to 160°C/Gas mark 3.

Line a 1 kg loaf tin with greaseproof paper. Mix together all the ingredients adding more water if necessary and turn into the tin. Bake for 1 hour until firm to the touch.

This recipe may also be used for burgers and stuffing.

Quinoa nut roast

Good for: Preliminary Diet

Serves 6 to 8

225 g quinoa, cooked
125 g carrots, grated
125 g courgettes, grated
2 sticks celery, chopped
125 g ground almonds
50 g whole almonds, chopped
125 g sunflower seeds
4 tbsp olive oil
125 ml vegetable stock or mineral water
2 tbsp sago flour
fresh sage or tarragon, chopped or 1 tsp dried
sea salt

Preheat the oven to 160°C/Gas mark 3.

Line one or two loaf tins with greaseproof paper. Mix all the ingredients together and turn into the tins. Bake for 1 hour. A soup may be used as a sauce.

Apricot and almond pilaff

Good for: Preliminary Diet; Rotation Diet, Day 3;
Elimination Diet, Day 8

Serves 4

2 cups sorghum/quinoa (use quinoa on Rotation Diet, Day 3)
2 litres mineral water (sorghum) or 1 litre mineral water (quinoa)
sea salt
175 g fresh apricots, cut into quarters
125 g almonds
25 g sunflower seeds, for garnishing
2 tbsp sunflower oil

Rinse the sorghum and place in a saucepan with the water and a pinch of salt. Bring to the boil and simmer for 1 hour (30 minutes for quinoa) until soft adding the apricots during the last 5 minutes of cooking time. Cut the almonds in half, lengthways and add the sorghum, together with the tarragon. Serve, garnished with the sunflower seeds and pour over the sunflower oil.

Tempeh or tofu stir-fry

Good for: Rotation Diet, Day 3

Serves 4

225 g mangetout, topped and tailed
225 g green beans, sliced
125 g mung bean sprouts
2 heads chicory, sliced
275 g tempeh or tofu, cut into cubes
1 tbsp Tamari soya sauce
2 tbsp sunflower oil
50 g almonds, cut lengthways, for garnishing

Heat a little water in a wok and cook the vegetables in order of cooking time. Add the tempeh or tofu and soya sauce. Stir in the oil and garnish with almonds.

Vegetable goulash with dumplings

Good for: Elimination Diet, Day 12

Serves 4

225 g tomatoes, skinned and chopped

125 g French beans, cut into 2.5-cm lengths

125 g potatoes, cut into even-sized chunks

2 carrots, sliced

2 sticks celery

500 ml water

1 tbsp tomato purée

sprig of rosemary or thyme

sea salt or kelp

2 tbsp sunflower oil

FOR THE BARLEY DUMPLINGS

(see page 193)

Place all the vegetables and the water, in a heavy-based saucepan and bring to the boil. Add the tomato purée, seasoning and dumplings and cook gently for 40 minutes. Remove the sprigs, stir in the oil and serve.

Smoked tofu and mushroom kebabs

Good for: Elimination Diet, Day 13

Serves 4

225 g button mushrooms

4 wooden skewers

275 g smoked tofu

fresh herbs, for garnishing

French dressing (see page 197)

Cut the mushrooms into halves and use them raw or quickly blanched in boiling water. Cut the tofu into 2.5-cm cubes and thread onto a skewer alternating each cube with a mushroom. Arrange on a serving dish on a bed of lettuce leaves and pour over the salad dressing.

Green pepper and pine nut pizza

Good for: Elimination Diet, Day 12

Serves 4

FOR THE DOUGH

225 g barley flour (or rice flour)

225 g swede, cooked and mashed

125 ml olive oil

sea salt

FOR THE SAUCE

1 onion, peeled and chopped

1 garlic clove, peeled and chopped

225 g fresh tomatoes, skinned and chopped

1 courgette, grated

1 large green pepper, deseeded and sliced

2 tbsp tomato purée

sea salt

FOR THE TOPPING

50 g pine nuts

6 black olives stoned and halved

1 tsp oregano

Preheat the oven to 160°C/Gas mark 3.

To prepare the dough, mix together all the ingredients and mould into four individual rounds or press into a well-oiled rectangular baking tray.

For the sauce, cook the onion and garlic for 3 to 4 minutes until soft. Add the tomatoes, courgette, green pepper, tomato purée and salt and spoon onto the dough bases.

Top with pine nuts and olives and sprinkle with oregano. Bake for 20 to 25 minutes.

Breadfruit with ginger and green peppers

Good for: Elimination Diet, Day 14

Serves 4

1 breadfruit

2 green peppers, sliced

1 large pear, peeled, cored and sliced

3 cardamom pods, crushed

1 tsp ginger, grated

500 ml water

1 tbsp tahini

Peel and core the breadfruit and cut into chunks. Steam for 30 minutes until tender.

For the sauce, put the peppers and pear in a pan with the cardamom pods, ginger and water and cook until soft. Add the tahini and liquidise until smooth. Place the breadfruit on a serving dish and pour over the sauce.

Cashew nut and celery flan

Good for: Rotation Diet, Day 1

Serves 4

FOR THE PASTRY

4 tbsp sesame seed oil

225 g wheat or barley flour

water to mix

pinch of salt

FOR THE SAUCE

600 ml cashew nut milk, or vegetable stock

50 g wheat or barley flour

sea salt

FOR THE FILLING

4 sticks celery, diced and cooked

125 g cashew nuts

2 tbsp parsley, freshly chopped

Preheat the oven to 160°C/Gas mark 3.

For the pastry, rub the oil into the flour and form into a firm dough with a little water and a pinch of salt. Roll out the pastry and line a 20-cm flan dish. Bake blind (cover with greaseproof paper and weighed with baking beans) for 25 minutes until the pastry is evenly cooked.

For the sauce, heat the cashew nut milk/stock in a saucepan. Mix the flour with a little cold water and stir into the milk and stir briskly until the sauce thickens. Season to taste.

For the filling, spread the celery and cashew nuts evenly over the pastry and sprinkle with parsley. Pour over the sauce and bake for a further 25 minutes.

Green pepper and aubergine flan

Good for: Elimination Diet, Day 16; Rotation Diet, Day 2

Serves 4

FOR THE PASTRY CASE

125 g fine oatmeal

175 g cooked mashed potato

125 ml olive oil

pinch of salt

FOR THE FILLING

2 aubergines, thinly sliced

sea salt

2 green peppers, thinly sliced

8-10 pitted olives (optional)

FOR THE SAUCE

250 ml vegetable stock or water

1 onion, finely chopped

1 tbsp cornflour

1 tbsp freshly chopped basil

sea salt

Preheat the oven to 160°C/Gas mark 3.

To prepare the flan case, mix together the ingredients using a little cold water to make a firm dough. Roll out between two sheets of greaseproof paper or tough polythene and mould into a 23-cm flan dish.

For the filling, sprinkle the sliced aubergines with salt and leave for 30 minutes. Drain and dry on kitchen paper (this removes the bitterness). Steam or boil in a little water for 3 to 5 minutes until just tender and arrange in the flan case with the green peppers and olives.

For the sauce, bring the stock/water to the boil and cook the onion until soft. Mix the cornflour with a little cold water and stir into the stock to thicken the sauce. Add the basil and salt and pour into the flan case. Bake for 40 minutes.

Spinach and lentil flan

Good for: Rotation Diet, Day 3

Serves 4

FOR THE RICE PASTRY

175 g rice flour

50 g soya or gram flour

125 ml sunflower seed oil

125 ml water

FOR THE FILLING

350 ml vegetable stock or water

175 g brown lentils, sprouted

sea salt

275 g spinach

½ tsp ground fenugreek

sunflower seeds, for garnishing

Preheat the oven to 160°C/Gas mark 3.

Mix together all the pastry ingredients. Unlike pastry made with wheat, this dough does not roll easily, so it is better to pat down evenly into a 23-cm flan dish that has been well oiled.

For the filling, bring the stock/water to the boil and add the lentils and salt. Cook for 20 to 25 minutes until the lentils form a purée. Wash the spinach, drain and cook it in its own juices in a covered pan. Drain, chop and mix with the lentils and ground fenugreek. Spread the mixture in the flan case and bake for 25 minutes. Garnish with a sprinkling of sunflower seeds.

Feta cheese and cabbage pie

Good for: Rotation Diet, Day 4

Serves 4

FOR THE PASTRY CASE

450 g sweet potato baked, skinned and mashed

125 g butter

125 g tapioca flour

FOR THE FILLING

125 g Feta sheep's or goat's cheese

225 g cabbage, finely shredded

Preheat the oven to 150°C/Gas mark 2.

For the pastry, mix together the sweet potato, butter and tapioca flour and form into a dough. Take two-thirds and press into a 23-cm ovenproof flan dish. Fill with layers of thinly sliced Feta cheese and finely shredded cabbage.

On a floured board using tapioca flour to stop sticking, roll out the remaining dough to fit the top. Bake for 45 minutes until the top is crisp.

Vegetable and lentil dal

Good for: Elimination Diet, Day 22

Serves 4

500 ml stock or water

125 g green lentils, sprouted

1 onion, chopped

1 pepper, deseeded and chopped

2 sticks celery

2 carrots, chopped

1 tsp ground cumin

1 tsp ground coriander

2 bay leaves

sea salt or kelp

Pour the stock/water into a saucepan and bring to the boil. Add the lentils, vegetables and seasoning and return to the boil. Simmer for 20 minutes until all the vegetables are tender. Remove the bay leaves and serve on a bed of millet or bulgur wheat.

Cauliflower and chick pea curry

Good for: Elimination Diet, Day 15

Serves 4

2 tbsp olive oil

1 large onion, sliced

1 tsp ginger, grated

2 cloves garlic, crushed

2 tsp curry powder (wheat free)

125 g creamed coconut

1 tbsp tomato purée

225 g potatoes, diced

1 litre vegetable stock or water

225 g chickpeas, sprouted and cooked

1 small cauliflower, broken into florets

1 green pepper, deseeded and sliced

2 sticks celery, chopped

1 tbsp lemon juice

sea salt

Warm the oil and a little water in a pan and gently cook the onions until transparent but not brown. Add the ginger, garlic and curry powder and cool fry for 1 to 2 minutes, then add the coconut, tomato purée stock and potatoes. Bring to the boil and simmer for 5 minutes. Add the remaining ingredients and cook for a further 15 minutes until the vegetables are tender.

Sweet potato and parsnip bakes

Good for: Elimination Diet, Day 23

Serves 4

450 g cooked sweet potato, mashed

225 g cooked parsnips, mashed

1 large onion, finely chopped

1 clove garlic, crushed

1 tsp ground mustard seed

1 tbsp fresh parsley, chopped

sea salt

1 tbsp sesame seeds, for coating

Preheat the oven to 160°C/Gas mark 3.

Mix together the ingredients and form into potato cakes. Roll in the sesame seeds and bake for 25 minutes.

Buckwheat pasta with broccoli and walnuts

Good for: Rotation Diet, Day 4

Serves 4

225 g buckwheat spaghetti or pasta spirals (wheat free)

675 g broccoli

sea salt

125 g walnuts, pre-soaked and chopped

2 tbsp walnut oil

50 g freshly grated Parmesan cheese or walnuts (optional)

Cook the pasta in plenty of boiling, salted water until al dente (tender without being too soft). Drain and keep warm on a serving dish.

Cut the florets from the broccoli and cut the stalks diagonally across to make oval shapes (the stalks may be discarded and used in soup if you wish). Add a sprinkling of salt and steam for 4 to 5 minutes until the florets turn a rich green, taking care not to over-cook. Add the cooked broccoli and the walnuts to the pasta and spoon over the oil. May be served with walnuts or grated Parmesan cheese.

Root vegetable crumble

Good for: Elimination Diet, Day 25

Serves 4

FOR THE FILLING

250 ml vegetable stock

450 g of the following vegetables, diced: yam/sweet potato, turnip, carrots, parsnip, swede

2 leeks, sliced (optional)

2 sticks celery, sliced

15-cm strip kombu seaweed

1 bay leaf

pinch of nutmeg

2 tsp arrowroot or cornflour

sea salt

FOR THE CRUMBLE

125 ml olive oil

125 g barley, rye or wheat flour

50 g chestnut flour

50 g sunflower seeds, chopped

50 g rolled oats

50 g hazelnuts, chopped

1 tbsp chopped parsley

sea salt

Preheat the oven to 160°C/Gas mark 3.

For the filling, pour the stock into a saucepan. Bring to the boil and add the vegetables and seasoning. Return to the boil and then cover and simmer until tender. Mix the arrowroot with a little cold water and add to the vegetables to thicken the juices. Remove the bay leaf and place the vegetable mixture in an ovenproof dish.

Make the crumble by lightly working the oil into the flour with your fingertips. Add the seeds, nuts, oats and parsley, season and mix together. Sprinkle over the vegetables and bake for 25 to 30 minutes.

Kedgeree

Good for: Elimination Diet, Day 26

Serves 4

1 large onion, peeled and chopped

2 cloves garlic, crushed

1 tsp ginger, mashed, or ½ tsp ground ginger

1 green pepper, deseeded and chopped

450 g cooked flaked cod, haddock or other saltwater fish

175 g wholemeal rice, cooked

2 tsp turmeric

juice of 1 lemon

sea salt or kelp

2 tbsp sesame seed oil

1 tbsp freshly chopped parsley, for garnishing

Gently cook the onion, garlic, ginger and pepper in a little water until soft. Stir in the fish, rice and seasonings and when thoroughly mixed and cooked through, turn onto a serving dish. Stir in the oil and garnish with parsley.

Millet croquettes

Good for: Rotation Diet, Day 1

Serves 4

225 g millet, cooked

3 sticks celery, diced

3 carrots, grated

2 tbsp millet flour

1 to 2 tbsp tahini

1 tbsp fresh parsley, chopped

125 ml water

sea salt or kelp

25 g sesame seeds, for coating

Preheat the oven to 150°C/Gas mark 2.

Mix together all the ingredients and form into croquettes. Roll in the sesame seeds and bake for 25 minutes.

Baked beans in tomato sauce

Good for: Elimination Diet, Day 20

Serves 4

225 g haricot beans, soaked and sprouted

1 carrot, diced

1 stick celery, diced

1 onion, chopped

1 clove garlic, crushed

225 g tomatoes skinned, deseeded and chopped

1 tbsp tomato purée

600 ml game stock or water

1 tsp ground cumin

1 tbsp chopped parsley

sea salt

Preheat the oven to 160°C/Gas mark 3. Place all the ingredients in a casserole dish and bake in the oven for 1½ hours.

Stuffed baked potatoes

Good for: Elimination Diet, Days 15 & 28

Serves as many as you like

baked potatoes

FOR THE FILLINGS

fromage frais, celery and chives

Cheddar cheese, mushrooms (chopped and cooked) and thyme

tuna fish with sweetcorn relish

salmon and tomato relish

Cheddar cheese and chutney

Preheat the oven to 190°C/Gas mark 5.

Scrub the potatoes and prick all over with a fork. Bake for about 1 hour until tender. Remove from the oven, cut a cross in the top, press open and scoop out some of the soft centre, placing it in a bowl. Mash with a filling and pile the mixture back into the potato and return to the oven for a further 10 minutes to heat through.

Mixed vegetable terrine

Good for: Rotation Diet, Day 1

Serves 4

350 g carrots

350 g parsnips

350 g celeriac

3 tsp barley or wheat flour

3 tbsp sesame seed oil

sea salt

2 tbsp freshly chopped parsley

2 sheets nori seaweed

Preheat the oven to 160°C/Gas mark 3 and line the base of a 1.4 kg loaf tin.

Cook the vegetables in separate saucepans and allow to cool. Blend each one separately in a blender adding 1 tsp of flour, 1 tbsp of oil and a pinch of salt to each. Blend the parsley with the celeriac.

Carefully spoon the purées into the loaf tin starting with a parsnip layer, then the carrot and finally the celeriac, placing a sheet of nori seaweed between each layer. Bake for 1½ hours until firm. Cool and then refrigerate. Turn out of the tin when cold.

Polenta with tomato and pepper sauce

Good for: Rotation Diet, Day 2

Serves 4

6 fresh tomatoes, skinned and chopped

1 pepper, deseeded and diced

2 spring onions, chopped

1 clove garlic, crushed

1 tsp basil

½ tsp cayenne pepper

sea salt

FOR THE POLENTA

(see page 86)

Cook the vegetables and seasonings in a little water for 15 minutes, until tender. Rub through a sieve or leave chunky. Cut the polenta into 5-cm squares. Serve hot with the tomato sauce.

Artichoke and three-bean casserole

Good for: Rotation Diet, Day 3

Serves 4

600 ml vegetable stock or water

175 g fresh French beans, cut into thirds

6 to 8 Jerusalem or globe artichoke hearts

175 g kidney beans, sprouted and cooked

175 g black-eyed beans, sprouted and cooked

½ tsp nutmeg

1 tbsp fresh tarragon or 2 tsp umeboshi purée

sea salt

Bring the stock/water to the boil and cook the French beans and artichoke hearts until tender. Add the remaining ingredients and flavourings and simmer for a further 10 to 15 minutes.

Jerusalem artichokes may be used instead of globe artichokes.

Spinach roulade with chickpea and salsify filling

Good for: Rotation Diet, Day 3

Serves 4

250 g spinach

4 eggs separated

50 g rice flour

sea salt

FOR THE FILLING

450 g salsify

225 g chickpeas, sprouted and cooked

sea salt

Preheat the oven to 170°C/Gas mark 3 and line a 33 x 22-cm Swiss roll tin with greaseproof paper and brush with oil.

Wash the spinach and discard the stalks. Cook in its own juice for 4 to 5 minutes until tender. Cool and drain well and place in a food mixer with the egg yolks, rice flour and salt and blend to form a smooth mixture. Whisk the egg whites in a clean bowl until they form stiff peaks. Fold into the spinach mixture and spread into the prepared tin. Cook for 20 minutes until firm.

For the filling, scrub the salsify and boil for 20 to 25 minutes. Peel and dice. Place in a food mixer with the cooked chickpeas and seasoning and blend until smooth adding some of the chickpea water to form a spreadable mixture. Turn the cooked roulade out on to a large sheet of greaseproof paper and peel off the lining paper. Spread with the chickpea filling and immediately roll up with the help of the paper. May be served hot or cold.

VEGETABLES AND ACCOMPANIMENTS

Rice

Good for: Preliminary Diet; Elimination Diet, Days 1-8

Serves 4

225 g organic wholegrain rice

pinch of sea salt

500 ml mineral water

Rinse the rice and place in a saucepan with the salt. Pour over the water and bring to the boil. Turn the heat down, place the lid on the saucepan and simmer gently for 30 minutes, until all the water has been absorbed. Do not rinse as this will wash away the nutrients. If there is too much water, strain and use the liquid in soup.

To cook pre-soaked rice discard the water that was used for soaking and follow the above procedure. The cooking time will be reduced to approximately 15 minutes.

Millet, quinoa or amaranth

Good for: Preliminary Diet; Elimination Diet, Days 1-8

Serves 4

Follow the method for rice, reducing the amount of water to 400 ml.

Sorghum

Good for: Preliminary Diet

Serves 4

225 g sorghum

1 litre mineral water

Cook as for rice, increasing the time to 1 hour.

Cardamom nut rice

Good for: Elimination Diet, Day 14

Serves 4

225 g organic long grain rice
1 onion, chopped
1 clove garlic, crushed
1 tsp fresh ginger, finely grated
3 black cardamom pods, crushed
½ tsp ground cumin
½ tsp ground lemongrass
½ tsp turmeric
sea salt
500 ml vegetable stock or water
2 tbsp olive oil
50 g pumpkin seeds
50 g cashew nuts
50 g almonds, blanched and halved lengthways
50 g sultanas

Put the rice in a pan with the onion, garlic, spices, salt and stock/water and bring to the boil. Cover and simmer for 25 to 30 minutes until the rice is cooked. Remove the cardamom pods from the rice and stir in the olive oil. Add the seeds, nuts and sultanas and serve.

Lentils

Good for: Preliminary Diet

Serves 4

400 g sprouted lentils
water
sea salt

Place the lentils in a saucepan with sufficient boiling water to cover, and a pinch of salt. Cook gently until tender. The cooking time will vary depending on how long the lentils have been sprouted.

Parsnip and walnut croquettes

Good for: Preliminary Diet; Elimination Diet, Day 7

Serves 4

225 g cooked parsnips

225 g cooked sweet potato or eddoe

2 sticks celery, finely diced

125 g walnuts, chopped

1 tsp tapioca flour

1 tbsp freshly chopped coriander

sea salt

1 tbsp millet flour, for coating

Preheat the oven to 160°C/Gas mark 3.

Mix together the ingredients and form into eight croquettes. Roll in millet flour and place on a baking tray and bake for 35 minutes.

Butternut squash with pine nuts

Good for: Elimination Diet, Day 10

Serves 4

675 g butternut squash, winter squash or marrow

sea salt

1 tsp ground cumin or seeds

1 tsp lemongrass

125 g pine nuts

sprigs of fresh mint, for garnishing

Peel the squash, cut in half lengthways, discard the seeds and cut into crosswise slices. Steam or cook with a little boiling water, sprinkling in the salt, cumin and lemongrass. Cook for 4 to 5 minutes until just tender. Arrange in a large shallow dish, in overlapping layers. Sprinkle over the pine nuts and garnish with mint. Serve hot or cold.

Brussels sprouts with chestnuts

Good for: Elimination Diet, Day 11

Serves 4

450 g whole cooked chestnuts or 225 g dried chestnuts, soaked and cooked

grated zest of 1 lemon

450 g Brussels sprouts

1 leek, sliced

1 tbsp olive oil

sea salt

1 tbsp chopped parsley, for garnishing

If you are using dried chestnuts, these will need to be soaked overnight before cooking. Cook the chestnuts and lemon zest in boiling salted water for 15 minutes until tender. Steam or boil the sprouts and leeks together with seasoning, for 5 to 7 minutes and drain. Add to the chestnuts and serve garnished with chopped parsley.

Stuffed papayas

Good for: Elimination Diet, Day 14

Serves 4

2 papayas

125 g trout (not farmed) or tofu

25 g pine nuts

50 g wild rice, cooked

juice of 1 lime

iceberg lettuce, for garnishing

alfalfa sprouts, for garnishing

Cut the papayas in half and discard the seeds. Flake the trout and mix with the pine nuts and wild rice. Spoon the mixture into the hollow centres and pour over the lime juice. Place on individual plates and garnish with iceberg lettuce and alfalfa sprouts.

Roasted Jerusalem artichokes

Good for: Rotation Diet, Day 3

Serves 4

600 g Jerusalem artichokes, washed and scrubbed

dripping

Preheat the oven to 170°C/Gas mark 3.

Place the artichokes in a roasting pan. Pour over a little dripping from cooking game or poultry. Roast for about 45 minutes until golden.

Broccoli with ginger and macadamia nuts

Good for: Elimination Diet, Day 27

Serves 4

450 g broccoli

1 tsp ginger, grated

50 g macadamia nuts, cut into slivers

Cut the broccoli into small pieces, separating the florets and cutting the stems into diagonal slices. Steam with the ginger for 3 to 4 minutes until soft but still bright green. Sprinkle with the nuts and serve with couscous or millet.

Greek style onions

Good for: Rotation Diet, Day 2

Serves 4

675 g small pickling onions

250 ml stock or water

1 tbsp olive oil

2 tsp tomato purée

sprig of fresh thyme

sea salt

Blanch the onions in boiling water for 1 minute only, then drain and rinse in cold water. Remove the skins with a small knife or your fingers. Place the onions in a heavy-based saucepan with the stock/water, oil, tomato purée, thyme and salt. Bring to the boil and simmer gently for 30 minutes. Remove the sprig of thyme and serve hot.

Baked vegetables

Good for: Rotation Diet, Day 2

Serves 4

1 red pepper, deseeded and halved

1 green pepper, deseeded and halved

1 large onion, skinned and quartered

6 whole cloves of garlic, skinned

3 to 4 courgettes, sliced lengthways

6 to 8 cherry tomatoes

1 bunch of asparagus, trimmed

2 tbsp olive oil or dripping

sea salt

herbs for garnishing, e.g. mint, basil, chives, oregano

Preheat the oven to 160°C/Gas mark 3.

Place the vegetables in a greased roasting pan with the oil or dripping and bake for 30 minutes. Sprinkle with salt and choice of herbs and serve hot.

Steamed vegetables

Good for: Preliminary Diet; Elimination Diet, Day 5

Serves 4

225 g broccoli florets

225 g swede, cut into julienne strips

225 g kohlrabi, diced

125 g turnip, diced

75 g radishes, sliced

75 g cabbage, shredded

sea salt

Using a steamer or just a small amount of water, cook vegetables in order of cooking time and season to taste. May be served with a sprinkling of flax seed oil.

Baked red cabbage

Good for: Elimination Diet, Day 25; Rotation Diet, Day 4

Serves 4

2 eating apples or pears

450 g red cabbage, shredded

4 to 5 cloves

½ tsp allspice

½ tsp mustard seeds

2 tbsp cider vinegar (optional)

Preheat the oven to 160°C/Gas mark 3.

Peel the apples and cut into small segments. Immerse quickly in salt water to prevent browning. Place in a casserole dish with the cabbage, spices and vinegar, if using, and bake for 1 hour. Remove the cloves and serve hot or cold.

Stuffed green peppers

Good for: Elimination Diet, Day 18

Serves 4

4 large green peppers
175 g minced lean lamb or sprouted and cooked aduki beans
175 g cooked rice
50 g chopped almonds
50 g chopped olives
1 onion, chopped
1 tomato, peeled and diced
1 tsp ground coriander seeds
½ tsp ground cinnamon
sea salt
450 ml stock

Preheat the oven to 180°C/Gas mark 4.

Prepare the peppers for stuffing by removing a piece from the top of each and scooping out the seeds. Mix together all the ingredients, except the stock, and stuff each of the peppers. Place in a baking dish, replace the tops of the peppers and pour over the stock. Bake for 1 hour, basting from time to time.

Bulgur wheat (cracked wheat)

Good for: Elimination Diet, Day 22

Serves 4

225 g bulgur wheat
pinch of salt
500 ml boiling water

Place the bulgur wheat in a bowl with the salt and pour over the boiling water. Leave for 15 to 20 minutes until all the water has been absorbed.

Bubble and squeak nests

Good for: Elimination Diet, Day 27; Rotation Diet, Day 4

Serves 4

450 g sweet potato or yam, grated

225 g cabbage, shredded

50 g butter

50 g amaranth or buckwheat flour

50 g grated cheese (optional)

Preheat the oven to 150°C/Gas mark 2.

Mix together the grated vegetables and bind with the butter and flour. Divide into four mounds on a well-greased baking sheet and shape into nests. Top with grated cheese, if using, and bake for 35 minutes.

Braised celery

Good for: Rotation Diet, Day 1

Serves 4

4 celery hearts, trimmed

2 tbsp sesame seed oil

25 g flour

300 ml stock or water

sea salt

Preheat the oven to 160°C/Gas mark 3.

Place the celery in a well-oiled casserole dish. Warm the oil in a pan, stir in the flour and cook for a few minutes. Gradually stir in the stock/water and cook until the sauce thickens, seasoning to taste. Pour over the celery and bake in the oven for 1 hour.

Barley dumplings

Good for: Elimination Diet, Day 12

Serves 4

225 g barley flour

1 tsp cream of tartar

½ tsp bicarbonate of soda

75 ml dripping or olive oil

Mix together the ingredients with a little cold water and mould into four dumplings.

Baked plantains

Good for: Rotation Diet, Day 2

Serves 4

4 medium plantains

Preheat the oven to 160°C/Gas mark 3.

Bake the plantains in their skins for 30 minutes.

Millet, hazelnut and tofu croquettes

Good for: Elimination Diet, Day 19

Serves 4

225 g millet flakes, cooked

275 g silken tofu

125 g ground hazelnuts

1 tbsp tamari soya sauce

1 tbsp chopped fresh parsley

sea salt

2 tbsp millet flour, for coating

Preheat the oven to 160°C/Gas mark 3.

Blend together all the ingredients and divide into eight croquettes. Roll in the millet flour and bake for 25 minutes.

Mustard sauce

Good for: Rotation Diet, Day 4

Serves 4

25 g butter

25 g tapioca flour

125 ml sheep's milk

1 tsp ground mustard

1 tbsp cider vinegar (optional)

sea salt

Melt the butter in a saucepan over gentle heat and stir in the flour to make a roux. Cook for 2 to 3 minutes, allowing it to bubble but not to change colour. Remove from the heat and gradually stir in the milk. Return to the heat, add the mustard, vinegar and salt and stir until the sauce thickens.

Mayonnaise

Good for: Elimination Diet, Day 15

Serves 4

2 quail's egg yolks

1 whole quail's egg

1 tbsp lemon juice

½ tsp ground mustard

pinch white pepper

sea salt

125 ml walnut oil, olive oil or mixture

Have all the ingredients at room temperature. Place the eggs, lemon juice and seasoning in a liquidiser and blend for a few seconds. Turn on to maximum speed and slowly pour in the oil until it thickens.

Tofu mayonnaise

Good for: Elimination Diet, Day 25; Rotation Diet, Day 3

Serves 4

225 g silken tofu

1 clove garlic, crushed (optional) (not for Day 3)

2 tbsp safflower or sunfower seed oil

2 tbsp cider vinegar (or wine vinigar for Day 3)

pinch of white pepper (not for Day 3)

sea salt to taste

Place all the ingredients in a liquidiser and blend until smooth.

Egg mayonnaise

Good for: Rotation Diet, Day 3

Serves 4

2 egg yolks at room temperature

2 tbsp wine vinegar

½ tsp sea salt

250 ml safflower oil at room temperature

Place all the ingredients in a liquidiser except for the oil and blend for 1 minute. Remove the top from the liquidiser, turn on to top speed and add the oil a few drops at a time until the mixture thickens.

Ginger syrup

Good for: Elimination Diet, Day 18

Serves 4

125 ml water

1 tsp grated ginger

500 ml white grape juice

Bring the water to the boil and add the ginger. Cook for 2 to 3 minutes and add to the grape juice. Continue cooking until the liquid is reduced by half. Strain and use hot or cold.

Tomato sauce

Good for: Elimination Diet, Day 19

Serves 4

450 g tomatoes, skinned, seeded and cut into chunks

2 sticks celery, chopped

1 clove garlic, crushed

4 spring onions, chopped

1 tbsp tomato purée

1 tbsp fresh basil, chopped

sea salt

2 tbsp sunflower/safflower oil

Gently cook the vegetables until soft. Add the tomato purée, basil and seasoning and cook for a further minute. Stir in the oil before serving but do not heat.

Redcurrant sauce

Good for: Preliminary Diet

Serves 4

225 g redcurrants

250 ml mineral water

1 tbsp fruit sugar, honey or maple syrup

2 tsp sago or tapioca flour

Place the redcurrants in a saucepan with the water. Bring to the boil and simmer until cooked. Add the sugar and thicken with the sago/tapioca flour mixed with a little cold water.

Horseradish sauce

Good for: Rotation Diet, Day 4

Serves 4

1 small dessert apple, peeled and cored

175 g turnip, diced

1 tsp ground lemongrass

½ tsp ground mustard seed

sea salt

2 tsp tapioca flour, for thickening

75 g fresh horseradish, grated

Cook the apple and turnip in a little water until tender. Cool slightly and purée in a liquidiser with the seasonings. Return to the saucepan, reheat and use a little tapioca flour to thicken. Stir in the grated horseradish and serve.

SALADS AND DRESSINGS

French dressing

Good for: Elimination Diet, Day 11

Serves 4

juice of 2 lemons

125 ml cold pressed virgin olive oil/walnut oil

1 tsp ground mustard

1 clove garlic, crushed

1 tsp fresh mint, chopped

½ tsp sea salt

Combine all the ingredients in a jar and shake well.

Salad dressing

Good for: Rotation Diet, Day 1

Serves 4

juice of 2 lemons

4 tbsp oil (wheat germ oil and/or sesame seed oil)

1 tbsp tahini (optional)

½ tsp sea salt, black pepper

Combine all the ingredients in a jar and shake well.

Fresh green salad

Good for: Rotation Diet, Day 4

Serves 4

Chinese leaves

watercress

mustard and cress

shredded cabbage

sorrel leaves

Mix together any or all of the leaves and served with salad dressing.

Fresh winter salad

Good for: Rotation Diet, Day 4

Serves 4

grated raw swede

kohlrabi

turnips

sliced radishes

water chestnuts

shredded white cabbage

red dessert apple, cut into segments

Mix together the ingredients and serve with a dressing or mustard sauce.

Fennel and bean sprout salad

Good for: Preliminary Diet; Elimination Diet, Day 25

Serves 4

1 large fennel, thinly sliced

225 g bean sprouts

½ cucumber, sliced

1 courgette, diced

125 g seedless green grapes

1 nectarine, cut into segments

4 Chinese leaves, shredded

Arrange the ingredients on a bed of shredded Chinese leaves and serve with fresh mayonnaise or salad dressing, which may be made with cider vinegar.

Arame with sesame seeds

Good for: Preliminary Diet; Elimination Diet, Day 16

Serves 4

125 g dried and shredded arame

1 carrot, cut into matchsticks

50 g sesame seeds

Rinse the arame seaweed and place in a pan with enough cold water to cover and leave to soak for 10 minutes. Add the carrot and bring to the boil and simmer for 30 minutes until all the water has been absorbed. Turn into a serving dish. Sprinkle the sesame seeds on the top.

Melon, cucumber and strawberry salad

Good for: Elimination Diet, Day 10

Serves 4

1 small lettuce, shredded

1 honeydew melon, cut into cubes

½ cucumber, cut in half and sliced

225 g strawberries, sliced

pumpkin seeds

cold pressed olive oil

sprigs of fresh mint, for garnishing

Place the shredded lettuce on a serving dish and arrange the other ingredients on top. Sprinkle with oil and garnish with mint.

Egg and pasta salad

Good for: Elimination Diet, Day 11

Serves 4

250 g buckwheat spirals

2 tsp olive oil

125 g celeriac, cut into strips and blanched

3 sticks celery, sliced

125 g asparagus tips

50 g walnuts

6 to 8 quail eggs, hard boiled and cut in half

1 tbsp dill, for garnishing

Cook the buckwheat in boiling water until al dente adding a little oil to the water to prevent sticking. Drain and allow to cool on a serving dish. Add the celeriac, celery, asparagus tips and walnuts and arrange the eggs on the top. Pour over a little French dressing and garnish with dill.

Coleslaw

Good for: Elimination Diet, Day 15

Serves 4

2 red apples, cored and diced

1 tbsp lemon juice

1 small white cabbage, shredded

225 g grated carrot

2 sticks celery, sliced

1 tbsp chopped chives

75 g raisins

2 tbsp mayonnaise

chopped fresh parsley, for garnishing

Toss the apple in lemon juice to prevent browning. Mix together all the dry ingredients, stir in the mayonnaise and sprinkle with parsley.

Rice, barley and bean sprout salad

Good for: Elimination Diet, Day 17

Serves 4

175 g cooked rice

50 g cooked pot barley

175 g French beans, sliced and cooked

125 g garden peas, cooked

125 g bean sprouts

2 spring onions, chopped (optional)

salad dressing

4 heads of chicory or 1 bunch of watercress, for garnishing

Allow the cooked grains and vegetables to cool. Mix in with the remaining ingredients and pour over the salad dressing. Place in the centre of a serving dish and arrange chicory leaves or watercress around the edge.

Prawn, avocado and fennel salad with buckwheat pasta

Good for: Elimination Diet, Day 18

Serves 4

225 g buckwheat pasta

salad leaves

350 g peeled prawns

2 ripe avocado pears, sliced

1 bulb fennel, sliced

salad dressing (see page 198)

1 tsp dill

sprigs of thyme, for garnishing

6 to 8 black olives, for garnishing

Cook the pasta until al dente. Drain and allow to cool. Arrange the salad leaves on a serving dish and place the prawns, avocado pears, fennel and buckwheat pasta on top. Spoon over the salad dressing, sprinkle with dill and garnish with sprigs of thyme and black olives.

Couscous salad

Good for: Elimination Diet, Day 27

Serves 4

225 g couscous

600 ml boiling water

2 tomatoes, skinned and diced

1 small green pepper, deseeded and diced

2 spring onions, finely sliced

juice of 1 lemon

freshly chopped basil or mint

sea salt and black pepper

Rinse the couscous in a fine mesh strainer. Place in a bowl and pour on the hot water. Allow to stand for 15 minutes until the water has been absorbed. When cool, mix with the vegetables, herbs and seasoning.

Greek salad

Good for: Elimination Diet, Day 20

Serves 4

1 small cos lettuce

2 heads of chicory

4 tomatoes, halved and sliced

½ cucumber, diced lengthways

1 small red pepper

1 small green pepper

125 g pitted black olives

125 g ewe's milk Feta cheese, cut into cubes

French dressing (see page 197)

1 tsp oregano, for garnishing

Bunch the lettuce leaves together and cut into thin strips with a sharp knife. Place on the bottom of a serving dish and arrange the other ingredients on top. Spoon over the dressing and sprinkle with oregano.

Orange and fennel salad

Good for: Rotation Diet, Day 1

Serves 4

4 heads of fennel, sliced

2 large oranges, peeled and divided into segments

1 tbsp sprouted fennel seeds (optional)

2 to 3 sprigs of fennel leaf, for garnishing

salad dressing

Mix together all the ingredients and pour over the dressing.

Avocado sweet and sour salad

Good for: Elimination Diet, Day 23

Serves 4

FOR THE DRESSING

juice of 1 lemon

2 tbsp sweet almond oil

ground ginger

salt and black pepper

julienne strips of orange peel, for garnishing

2 avocado pears, cut into chunks

lemon juice

225 g carrots, finely shredded

225 g mung bean sprouts

juice of 2 oranges, 2 oranges, divided into segments

50 g organic sultanas

Make the dressing by mixing together all the ingredients. Sprinkle the avocado pear with lemon juice to stop browning. Mix together all the salad items in a salad bowl and pour over the dressing.

Cucumber, avocado and asparagus salad

Good for: Rotation Diet, Day 2

Serves 4

2 avocados

125 g asparagus tips

1 cucumber, cut into chunks

paprika pepper

sprig of mint, for garnishing

Cook the asparagus tips in a little water until just tender. Drain and allow to cool. Cut the avocados into half segments, removing the skin and stone. Mix with the cucumber and asparagus and sprinkle with paprika pepper and garnish with mint.

Mixed grain salad

Good for: Rotation Diet, Day 1

Serves 4

125 g cooked wheat barley or rye grains

125 g cooked millet

50 g cashew nuts, roughly chopped

sprouted seeds, e.g. dill, celery, aniseed

2 sticks celery, diced

50 g grated carrot

salad dressing

1 tbsp sesame seeds, for garnishing

freshly chopped parsley, for garnishing

Mix together all the ingredients keeping the sesame seeds and parsley for garnishing. Pour over the salad dressing. The grains may also be used, sprouted.

Green bean salad

Good for: Rotation Diet, Day 3

Serves 4

450 g French beans, cut in halves

sea salt

cold pressed safflower or sunflower seed oil

1 hard boiled egg, sieved

175 g alfalfa sprouts

Place the beans in a saucepan with a pinch of salt and enough boiling water to cover. Cook for 7 to 10 minutes until tender. Drain well and toss in a little oil. Place in the middle of a serving dish and sprinkle with the sieved egg. Place the alfalfa sprouts around the edge of the dish. The egg may be replaced with chopped walnuts.

Seafood salad

Good for: Rotation Diet, Day 1

Serves 4

225 g pasta spirals, wheat, rye, barley or millet
450 g mussels
8 to 10 baby squid tentacles, cut from the bodies
225 g peeled prawns
salad dressing
2 tbsp freshly chopped parsley, for garnishing

To cook the pasta, fill a large saucepan with water and bring to the boil. Add the pasta and a pinch of salt. Cook until just tender, for 8 to 10 minutes according to the type of pasta used.

To prepare the mussels, pull off the beards and thoroughly wash and scrub the shells. Place in a shallow pan and cover with boiling water. Cook for 5 minutes, shaking the pan now and then. Remove the mussels as soon as the shells open and discard any that do not open.

Place the squid pieces in the mussel water and cook for 15 minutes until tender. Add the prawns and cook for a further 5 minutes. Drain and allow to cool. Cut the squid into rings and mix altogether with the mussels, prawns and cooked pasta.

Arrange on a serving dish and pour over the salad dressing and sprinkle with chopped parsley.

Cherry and almond salad

Good for: Rotation Diet, Day 3

Serves 4

350 g black cherries

1 nectarine

1 little gem or cos lettuce

125 g almonds, blanched

cold pressed, unrefined safflower or sunflower seed oil

Wash and stone the cherries, reserving a few with stalks for garnishing. Wash the nectarine and cut into small segments. Arrange the lettuce leaves around the edge of the plate and pile the fruit on top with the almonds. Sprinkle with oil and garnish with the whole cherries.

Pear and watercress salad

Good for: Rotation Diet, Day 4

Serves 4

4 ripe pears

1 bunch watercress, washed

2 tbsp cold pressed walnut oil

½ tsp ground mustard seeds

Peel and quarter the pears and quickly immerse them in salt water to prevent browning. Arrange in a serving bowl with the watercress and spoon over the oil and sprinkle with mustard seed.

BREADS, CAKES AND BISCUITS

Barley scone bread

Good for: Elimination Diet, Days 10 & 12

Serves 4

175 g barley flour

4 tbsp olive oil

50 g cashew nuts, chopped (optional)

1 tsp bicarbonate of soda

4 tbsp water

sea salt

Preheat the oven to 160°C/Gas mark 3.

Mix together all the ingredients and make into a large scone. Divide into 4 pieces. Bake for 20 to 25 minutes.

Corn bread

Good for: Elimination Diet, Day 16; Rotation Diet, Day 2

Serves 4

175 g maize flour

125 g cooked squash or pumpkin

1 tsp cream of tartar

½ tsp bicarbonate of soda

4 tbsp olive oil

125 ml water

2 tsp honey (fruit sugar for Day 2)

Preheat the oven to 150°C/Gas mark 2 and line a loaf tin with greaseproof paper.

Mix together all the ingredients and bake for 40 to 45 minutes until firm.

Rice bread

Good for: Preliminary Diet

Serves 4

125 g rice flakes

425 ml mineral water

125 g pea or lentil flour

125 g almonds or brazil nuts, ground

125 g kohlrabi, grated or turnip

2 tbsp sesame seed oil or olive oil

1 tbsp tapioca flour or arrowroot

1 tsp cream of tartar

½ tsp bicarbonate of soda

½ tsp sea salt

Preheat the oven to 150°C/Gas mark 2 and line a loaf tin with greaseproof paper.

Pour the water onto the rice flakes to soften. Mix all the ingredients, transfer to the loaf tin and bake for 1 hour, until firm.

Raisin bun loaf

Good for: Preliminary Diet; Rotation Diet, Day 3

Serves 4

For the Preliminary Diet follow the recipe for rice bread and add 125 g raisins.

For Rotation Diet follow the recipe for rice and sago bread and add 125 g raisins.

Rice and sago bread

Good for: Preliminary Diet; Rotation Diet, Day 3

Serves 4

125 g sago pearls

375 ml mineral water

125 g rice flour

50 g lentil flour

1 tsp cream of tartar

½ tsp bicarbonate of soda

Preheat the oven to 150°C/Gas mark 2 and line a loaf tin with greaseproof paper.

Pour the water onto the sago and leave to soak for 30 minutes to soften. Mix with the remaining ingredients, transfer to the loaf tin and bake for 45 minutes.

Soda bread

Good for: Rotation Diet, Day 1

Serves 4

450 g permissible flour

1 tsp bicarbonate of soda

½ tsp salt (optional)

250 ml water or nut milk

Preheat the oven to 170°C/Gas mark 3.

Mix together all the ingredients and form into a firm dough. Shape into a flat round loaf, cut a deep cross on top and bake for 40 minutes until firm.

Rye bread

Good for: Elimination Diet, Day 20; Rotation Diet, Day 1

Serves 4

40 g fresh yeast

1 tsp raw cane molasses sugar

250 ml warm water

½ tsp salt

450 g rye flour

1 tsp caraway seeds

Mix the yeast with the sugar and pour on half the water. Leave for 5 to 10 minutes for it to froth. Add the salt to the flour and pour in the yeast mixture. Add the caraway seeds and the remaining water and mix to a dough. Knead for 5 to 10 minutes and then leave covered in a warm place until it has doubled in size. Knock back and knead again for 2 to 3 minutes. Form into two round loaves and place on a well-greased baking tray. Cover and leave for 30 minutes until well risen. Preheat the oven to 200°C/Gas mark 6.

Bake the loaves for 10 minutes at 200°C/Gas mark 6, then reduce the oven setting to 180°C/Gas mark 4 and bake for a further 25 minutes.

Russian-style rye bread can be made with just rye flour, water and salt. Wholemeal wheat or spelt wheat bread can be made following the above recipe but substituting the wheat flour for rye and reducing the quantity of yeast to 25 g. Omit the caraway seeds and use cashew nuts or a few wheat flakes instead. Sprinkle with sesame seeds, poppy seeds or wheat flakes.

Sprouted grain bread

Good for: Elimination Diet, Day 27; Rotation Diet, Day 1
Serves 4
450 g organic wheat grains
filtered water for sprouting
sea salt

Rinse the grains and leave to soak for 15 hours. Drain off the water and leave to sprout for two to three days until the grains have developed 2.5-cm sprouts, rinsing morning and evening.

Preheat the oven to 130°C/Gas mark ½. Place the grains in a meat mincer and grind the sprouts to a fine texture. Add the salt and place in a well-oiled loaf tin and bake for 4 to 5 hours, until the bread leaves the sides of the tin.

Buckwheat chappatis

Good for: Elimination Diet, Day 23; Rotation Diet, Day 4
Serves 4
175 g buckwheat flour
water

Mix the flour with enough water to make a firm dough. Break off small pieces and roll out into very thin rounds. Cook in a dry frying pan until brown, then grill under a hot grill until they puff up.

Pitta bread

Good for: Rotation Diet, Day 1

Serves 4

25 g fresh or dried yeast

1 tsp unrefined molasses sugar

250 ml warm water

1 tsp salt

450 g organic strong whole wheat flour or barley flour

FOR THE HERB AND SESAME TOPPING (OPTIONAL)

sesame seed oil

2 tbsp chopped fresh parsley or coriander leaves

2 tbsp sesame seeds

Mix the yeast, sugar and water and leave in a warm place for 5 to 10 minutes until frothy. Mix the salt with the flour and combine with the yeast liquid to form a soft dough. Knead for 10 minutes. Place in a large oiled polythene bag and leave in a warm place until doubled in size. Preheat the oven to 220°C/Gas mark 7.

On a floured board, knead the dough for a minute and divide into eight portions. Knead each portion into a small ball and roll out into an oval shape and lay these onto several oiled baking trays. Cover with oiled polythene and leave to rest for 30 minutes.

Brush with sesame seed oil and sprinkle with herbs and sesame seeds. Bake for 8 minutes until risen and puffed.

Celebration carrot cake

Good for: Elimination Diet, Day 28

Serves 4

175 g wholemeal flour

125 g shredded carrot

250 ml crushed pineapple and juice

125 g coconut

125 g walnuts, chopped

3 eggs, beaten

1 tsp cream of tartar

½ tsp bicarbonate of soda

125 g butter or oil

2 tsp cinnamon

2 tsp natural vanilla essence

Preheat the oven to 150°C/Gas mark 2 and line and grease a cake tin.

Mix together all the ingredients, transfer to the cake tin and bake for 40 minutes.

Pineapple upside-down cake

Good for: Rotation Diet, Day 2

Serves 4

1 pineapple, sliced

175 g maize flour

175 g cornflour

125 g corn syrup

125 ml olive oil

500 ml water

1 tsp bicarbonate of soda

Preheat the oven to 160°C/Gas mark 3. Put the sliced pineapple into the bottom of a well-oiled ovenproof dish. Mix together the other ingredients and pour onto the fruit. Cook for 45 minutes until firm.

Rich fruit cake

Good for: Rotation Diet, Day 3

Serves 4

6 tbsp oil (almond or sunflower)

50 to 125 g unrefined sugar or honey

6 free-range eggs

275 g rice flour

½ tsp bicarbonate of soda

1 tsp cream of tartar

1 tsp nutmeg

675 g mixed organic dried fruit, e.g. raisins, sultanas, currants, dried cherries,
  prunes, apricots

125 g chopped almonds

Preheat the oven to 150°C/Gas mark 2 and line a 22-cm cake tin with greaseproof paper.

Cream the oil with the sugar or honey and add the beaten eggs. Add the cream of tartar and bicarbonate of soda and nutmeg to the flour and fold into the mixture with the fruit and almonds. Bake for 1½ to 2 hours. Leave to cool in the tin for 6 to 8 hours.

Cooked and puréed dried apricots may be used in this recipe as an alternative to eggs: use 1 tbsp of purée for one egg.

Sticky prune cake

Good for: Rotation Diet, Day 3

Serves 4

125 g prunes

3 free-range eggs

125 g rice flakes

250 ml water

125 ml almond oil

1 tbsp honey

1 tsp cream of tartar

½ tsp bicarbonate of soda

50 g chopped almonds, for the topping

Preheat the oven to 160°C/Gas mark 3 and line a shallow cake tin approximately 20-cm square.

Place the prunes in a saucepan with enough water to cover. Simmer for 10 minutes until tender. Drain, remove stones and cut into small pieces. Whisk the eggs until thick and stir in the prunes with the remaining ingredients. Pour the mixture into the cake tin, sprinkle the chopped almonds over the top and bake for 40 minutes until firm to the touch.

Carob and walnut/coconut brownies

Good for: Preliminary Diet

Serves 4

125 g dates, chopped

125 g brown rice flour

50 g carob powder

50 g green banana flour

125 g sultanas

125 g walnuts, roughly chopped

125 ml olive oil or sesame seed oil

250 ml mineral water

1 tsp cinnamon

Preheat the oven to 160°C/Gas mark 3 and grease a 27 x 18-cm flat baking tin. Soften the dates in a little hot water and then mix together all the ingredients. Turn into the baking tin and bake for 45 minutes. Allow to cool in the tin before cutting into squares.

Carob and coconut brownies

Good for: Rotation Diet, Day 3

Serves 4

125 g carob powder

175 g brown rice flour

125 g desiccated coconut

175 g dates soaked in 250 ml hot water

125 ml almond oil

2 to 4 tbsp honey

2 eggs beaten

Preheat the oven to 160°C/Gas mark 3 and grease a 27 x 18-cm flat baking tin.

Place all the ingredients in a bowl and mix well. Turn into the baking tin and bake for 45 minutes. Allow to cool in the tin before cutting into squares.

Barley muffins

Good for: Elimination Diet, Day 17

Serves 4

125 g brown rice flakes

250 ml soya milk

125 g barley flour

50 g sunflower seeds, chopped

50 g seedless raisins

2 tsp dried yeast

1 tsp fruit sugar

1 tsp arrowroot or sago flour

½ tsp cinnamon

Preheat the oven to 190°C/Gas mark 5 and line a loaf tin.

Soak the rice flakes in the soya milk to soften and then mix together all the ingredients and spoon into the loaf tin until two-thirds full. Leave in a warm place to rise for 30 minutes. Bake for 30 minutes until firm.

Date and coconut muesli bars

Good for: Elimination Diet, Day 16

Serves 4

225 g chopped dried dates

2 tbsp water

225 g rolled oats

225 g creamed coconut, warmed

125 ml sesame seed oil

grated zest of 1 orange (optional)

Preheat the oven to 160°C/Gas mark 3 and oil or line a baking tin.

Put the chopped dates and water in a pan and gently heat for 15 to 20 minutes until soft. Place in a food mixer and mix with the remaining ingredients. Turn into the baking tin and bake for 40 minutes. Allow to cool before cutting and transferring to a wire rack.

Apple and hazelnut muffins

Good for: Rotation Diet, Day 4

Serves 4

125 g hazelnuts, skinned and chopped

225 g sweet potato, baked, skinned and cooled

125 g buckwheat flour

1 large or 2 small eating apples, peeled and chopped

125 g butter

1 tbsp maple syrup (optional)

1 tsp allspice

Preheat the oven to 150°C/Gas mark 2 and grease 9 muffin tins.

To remove the skins from the hazelnuts, place in a grill pan and grill lightly for 2 to 3 minutes, watching carefully. Rub the nuts between two sheets of kitchen paper or in a clean tea towel and the skins will flake off.

Mix together all the ingredients and put into the muffin tins. Bake for 15 to 20 minutes.

Barley and cashew nut scones

Good for: Rotation Diet, Day 1

Serves 4

225 g barley flour

1 tsp bicarbonate of soda

125 g cashew nuts, ground or chopped

4 tbsp sesame seed oil

1 tsp sugar (optional)

250 ml water

Preheat the oven to 160°C/Gas mark 3.

Mix together the ingredients and form into a firm dough. Cut into individual scones with a pastry cutter or make one large scone, cutting a cross on the top. Bake for 10 to 15 minutes, according to size.

Green banana and oatmeal scones

Good for: Rotation Diet, Day 2

Serves 4

125 g green banana flour

125 g fine oatmeal

25 g fruit sugar

1 tsp bicarbonate of soda

2 tbsp olive oil

250 ml nut milk or water

Preheat the oven to 160°C/Gas mark 3.

Place the dry ingredients in a large bowl and rub in the oil. Add sufficient nut milk/water to form a firm dough. Roll out to about 2-cm thickness and cut into rounds with a 5-cm cutter. Bake for 10 to 15 minutes.

Buckwheat and chestnut dropped scones

Good for: Rotation Diet, Day 4

Serves 4

175 g buckwheat flour

125 g chestnut flour

600 ml water

Mix together the flours and the water. Drop in spoonfuls on to a hot griddle, dropping from the point of the spoon to keep the scone in good shape. Allow 1 dessertspoon for each scone or 1 tablespoon for larger ones. When bubbles appear and the scone is just beginning to brown on the underside, turn with a flat spatula and cook on the other side.

Delicious served with apple and pear spread, strawberry or raspberry sugarless jams, or with yoghurt, pecan nuts and maple syrup.

Carrot and fig slice

Good for: Rotation Diet, Day 1

Serves 4

175 g dried figs

175 g whole wheat flour

175 g grated carrot

75 ml sesame seed oil

½ tsp aniseed

Preheat the oven to 160°C/Gas mark 3 and grease or line an 18-cm baking tin.

Place the figs in a saucepan, cover with water and cook for 20 minutes. Drain and liquidise to a purée. Mix the purée with the rest of the ingredients and spoon into the baking tin and bake for 1 hour. Allow to cool before turning out.

Cherry and coconut slices

Good for: Rotation Diet, Day 3

Serves 4

125 g rice flakes soaked in 250 ml water

2 to 4 tbsp honey

4 tbsp almond oil

2 eggs beaten

50 g desiccated coconut

50 g dried cherries

Preheat the oven to 160°C/Gas mark 3 and oil or line a 20-cm baking tin.

Mix together all the ingredients and turn into the baking tin. Bake for 25 to 30 minutes until firm to the touch.

Orange and cashew nut crunchies

Good for: Rotation Diet, Day 1

Serves 4

4 tbsp sesame seed oil

125 g raw cane sugar or barley malt

225 g wholemeal flour

125 g ground cashew nuts

grated zest of 1 orange

Preheat the oven to 170°C/Gas mark 3 and grease a Swiss roll tin.

Warm the oil and cane sugar/barley malt in a saucepan for 2 to 3 minutes. Mix with the remaining ingredients and spoon into the Swiss roll tin and bake for 15 to 20 minutes. Allow to cool before cutting into fingers or squares.

Chocolate hazelnut biscuits

Good for: Elimination Diet, Day 26

Serves 4

225 g wheat flour or fine oatmeal

1 tsp cream of tartar

½ tsp bicarbonate of soda

125 g fruit sugar

50 g cocoa powder

1 tsp natural vanilla essence

50 g chopped hazelnuts, for decoration

Preheat the oven to 150°C/Gas mark 2 and line a baking sheet with greaseproof paper.

Mix together all the ingredients and divide into pieces the size of a walnut. Place on the lined baking sheet and flatten with a fork, dipped in cold water. Decorate with nuts. Bake for 25 to 20 minutes. Allow to cool before lifting on to a wire rack.

If using oatmeal, replace 1 tbsp with 1 tbsp tapioca or arrowroot flour.

Brazil nut cookies

Good for: Rotation Diet, Day 2

Serves 4

125 g fine oatmeal

50 g oatflakes

125 g Brazil nuts, finely chopped

75 g fruit sugar

4 tbsp olive oil

water to mix

1 tsp arrowroot or cornflour

Preheat the oven to 160°C/Gas mark 3 and grease a baking sheet.

Place all the dry ingredients in a large mixing bowl and rub in the oil. Add sufficient water to make a firm dough. Roll out on a surface dusted with arrowroot or cornflour and cut with a biscuit cutter. Place on the baking sheet and cook for 10 to 15 minutes, until light golden in colour.

DESSERTS

Fig and lime sorbet

Good for: Rotation Diet, Day 1

Serves 4

6 fresh figs

juice of 2 limes

cane sugar to taste

2 level tsp agar agar

FOR THE DECORATION

1 fresh fig, sliced thinly

julienne strips of lime

Wash and cut the figs into quarters and place in a saucepan. Bring to the boil, cover and gently cook for 5 minutes.

Allow to cool a little and liquidise, adding the lime juice, sugar and agar agar dissolved in a little hot water. Spoon into a freezer container and freeze for 1 to 2 hours until almost frozen. Return to the liquidiser and whip until light and fluffy. Return to the freezer until firm.

Scoop the ice cream to serve and decorate.

Blood oranges with cranberries

Good for: Rotation Diet, Day 1

Serves 4

4 blood oranges

zest of 1 orange

175 g cranberries

1 tbsp raw cane sugar

Cut the oranges into segments and the zest into julienne strips. Cook the cranberries for 2 to 3 minutes with the julienne strips and sugar. Allow to cool and then mix with the oranges. (May be enhanced with a little cinnamon from Day 2).

Chicory coffee ice cream

Good for: Rotation Diet, Day 3

Serves 4

2 eggs or soya egg substitute

125 g honey

50 ml almond oil

600 ml soya milk

2 tsp chicory coffee granules

125 g ground almonds, for the topping

Beat the eggs and blend with the remaining ingredients. Place in a shallow freezing tray and freeze until just beginning to set. Take out and whisk until light and fluffy. Return to the freezer. Serve with a topping of ground almonds.

Pistachio nut semolina with lime

Good for: Rotation Diet, Day 1

Serves 4

500 ml cashew nut milk

zest of 1 lime and juice of 2 limes

2 tbsp raw cane sugar

2 tbsp semolina

125 g unsalted pistachio nuts, chopped

Bring the cashew nut milk to the boil and add the zest of lime cut into julienne strips. Add the sugar and sprinkle in the semolina, stirring briskly until the mixture thickens. Cool and stir in the lime juice and chopped pistachio nuts, keeping a few for decoration.

Grilled pineapple with macadamia nuts

Good for: Rotation Diet, Day 2

Serves 4

1 large pineapple

1 tbsp fruit sugar

50 g macadamia nuts, sliced

Using a serrated knife, trim off about 1 cm from each end of the pineapple, saving some of the leaves. Cut into quarters lengthways and carefully trim away the core, then cut along the base of each quarter so the flesh is separated from the skin. Cut the flesh in half lengthways and then into four crossways to give bite-sized portions.

Sprinkle each quarter with fruit sugar and place under a grill until just beginning to caramelise. Decorate with macadamia nuts and serve.

Fruit crêpes

Good for: Rotation Diet, Day 2

Serves 4

125 g fine oatmeal, maize or quinoa flour

50 g cornflour or green banana flour

1 tsp fruit sugar

250 ml nut milk or water

Place all the dry ingredients in a bowl and add half the liquid. Beat well to form a smooth, thick batter. Gradually add the remaining liquid to produce a pouring consistency. Spoon 2 to 3 tbsp of the mixture on to a hot griddle and cook on both sides until just golden. Serve hot with a fruit filling of your choice.

Damson syllabub

Good for: Rotation Diet, Day 3

Serves 4

450 g damsons or plums

75 g unrefined beet sugar or honey

125 ml water

1 tbsp sago flour

2 egg whites

Wash the damsons/plums. Place the sugar in a saucepan with the water and stir over a gentle heat, until dissolved. Add the damsons, cover and simmer until soft. Mix the sago with a little cold water and stir into the damsons. Sieve into a large bowl, discard the stones and allow to cool.

Beat the egg whites until white and fluffy but not dry. Gently fold into the damsons and spoon the mixture into individual glass bowls.

Tapioca milk pudding

Good for: Rotation Diet, Day 4

Serves 4

75 g tapioca flakes

1 litre sheep's milk

1 tbsp maple syrup

knob of butter, sugarless jam or stewed or fresh fruit (optional)

Soak the tapioca in the milk for 1 hour. Gently simmer the tapioca in the milk, stirring from time to time, until cooked. Serve with a knob of butter, spoonful of sugarless jam or with stewed or fresh fruit.

Apricot and almond flan

Good for: Rotation Diet, Day 3

Serves 4

FOR THE RICE PASTRY

175 g rice flour

50 g soya flour

125 ml almond oil

125 ml water

FOR THE APRICOT FILLING

750 g apricots

250 ml water

1 to 2 tbsp honey (optional)

125 g ground almonds

50 g flaked or chopped almonds

Preheat the oven to 150°C/Gas mark 2 and oil a flan dish very thoroughly.

For the pastry, mix together all the ingredients. This dough does not roll easily, so it is better to pat down evenly into the flan dish.

For the filling, take half the apricots and place in a saucepan with the water and honey, if using. Bring to the boil and simmer until cooked. When cool, liquidise to a purée.

Make a layer of the ground almonds on top of the pastry base. Cut the remaining raw apricots into halves or slices and arrange on top of the ground almonds. Pour over the apricot purée and decorate the flan with the flaked almonds. Bake for 35 minutes.

Steamed apple pudding

Good for: Rotation Diet, Day 4

Serves 4

225 g sweet potato, baked, skinned and cooled

125 g buckwheat flour

2 large eating apples, peeled and chopped

125 g butter

1 tbsp concentrated apple juice

1 tsp ground cloves

Mix together all the ingredients. Butter a 1-litre bowl and pour in the mixture. Cover with a double layer of greaseproof paper. Steam in a saucepan of simmering water for 1 hour or for 30 minutes in a pressure cooker.

Bramble mousse

Good for: Rotation Diet, Day 4

Serves 4

450 g blackberries

125 ml water

3 tbsp concentrated apple juice

3 tbsp cold water

15 g powdered gelatine

125 ml double cream (or sheep's yoghurt)

Thoroughly wash the blackberries and place in a saucepan with the water and the apple concentrate to sweeten. Bring to the boil and simmer for 5 minutes until soft.

Put the cold water in a bowl and sprinkle on the gelatine and allow to stand for 3 minutes. Stir into the fruit and rub through a sieve to remove the pips and to make a purée. Allow to cool. Whisk the cream until it forms soft peaks and fold into the purée before it sets.

Pears in raspberry sauce

Good for: Rotation Diet, Day 4

Serves 4

500 ml water

4 firm but ripe pears, peeled

225 g raspberries

2 to 3 tbsp maple syrup

Put the water in a shallow pan and bring to the boil. Add the pears and poach for 10 to 12 minutes, until they look slightly translucent but still firm. Lift out into a serving dish and cook the raspberries in the poaching water for 2 to 3 minutes. Press the raspberries through a sieve to remove the pips, add the maple syrup to the juice and spoon this over the pears. May be served with crème fraîche or live yoghurt.

DRINKS AND DAIRY SUBSTITUTES

Lemon and orange barley water

Good for: Rotation Diet, Day 1

Serves 4

50 g pot barley

1 litre water

2 tbsp barley malt

2 oranges

1 lemon

Place the barley in a saucepan with the water. Bring to the boil and simmer for 1 hour. Stir in the barley malt and leave to cool.

Wash the fruit and grate the zest into a jug. Cut away the pith and discard. Thinly slice the flesh and add to the zest. Strain the barley water and pour into the jug with the fruit.

Lemon and elderflower cordial

Good for: Rotation Diet, Day 1

Serves 4

grated zest of 1 lemon and juice of 2 lemons

10 heads of freshly gathered elderflowers or 25 g dried elderflowers

2 tbsp raw cane sugar

1 litre boiling water

Place the lemon zest, elderflowers and sugar in a saucepan and pour on the boiling water. Leave for 10 to 20 minutes and strain off the juice. Add the fresh lemon juice and serve chilled with slices of lemon. Dilute to taste.

Elderberry punch

Good for: Rotation Diet, Day 1

Serves 4

900 g elderberries

500 ml water

zest and juice of 2 lemons

1 litre orange juice

500 ml green leaf tea, strained

2 tbsp grenadine (optional)

½ tbsp cane sugar or to taste

2 oranges, sliced

Place the elderberries in a large saucepan with the water and lemon zest and bring to the boil. Simmer for 10 minutes and then strain off the pulp. Pour the elderberry juice back into the saucepan and add the orange juice, lemon juice, tea and grenadine, if using. Add sugar to taste. Bring to the boil and then simmer for 10 minutes. Place slices of orange in a jug and pour on the punch. Serve hot.

This may be served chilled or as a hot punch with 2 sticks of cinnamon and 2 to 3 sprigs of thyme (from Rotation Diet, Day 2).

Strawberry yoghurt crush

Good for: Rotation Diet, Day 4

Serves 4

225 g strawberries, washed and hulled

225 g live sheep's yoghurt

2 tbsp maple syrup

250 ml water or cold lemongrass tea

ice cubes (optional)

Liquidise all the ingredients until smooth, adding the ice cubes, if using, a second or two at the end.

Rose hip cordial

Good for: Rotation Diet, Day 4

Serves 4

Gather well-ripened rose hips from the wild in the early autumn or from garden roses throughout the summer. Wash thoroughly and cut in half, lengthways. Place in a saucepan with enough water to float them and bring to the boil. Simmer gently for 30 minutes and strain. Sweeten with maple, concentrated apple/pear juice or rice syrup, according to taste and use in drinks. May be mixed with blackberries or raspberries.

Banana milk shake

Good for: Rotation Diet, Day 2

Serves 4

1 peeled banana

500 ml nut or oat milk

Place the ingredients in a liquidiser and blend until smooth. Serve immediately.

Tiger nut milk

Good for: Preliminary Diet; Elimination Diet, Day 7; Rotation Diet,
 Day 2

Serves 4

225 g tiger nuts washed and soaked over night

1 litre mineral water

Rinse the tiger nuts. Liquidise with the water and strain off the pulp.
Use poured over cereal and keep or freeze the pulp to use in recipes.

Oat milk

Good for: Elimination Diet, Day 16; Rotation Diet, Day 2

Serves 4

50 g oatmeal or flakes

1 litre water

1 tsp fruit sugar (optional)

drop of natural vanilla essence (optional)

Place the oats in a large pan with the water and bring to the boil.
Simmer for 10 minutes. Cool slightly, liquidise until smooth and
strain. Serve hot or cold but it is a particularly delicious and
warming drink served hot with a little sweetener.

Hemp seed milk

Good for: Rotation Diet, Day 2

Serves 4

125 g hemp seeds, soaked for 48 hours

1 litre water

Place the seeds in a pan with the water and bring to the boil. Simmer
for 15 to 20 minutes. Remove from the heat as soon as a yellow film
starts to form on the surface. Leave to cool for a few minutes and
then pour through a fine strainer or coffee filter. Serve chilled.

Rice milk

Good for: Preliminary Diet; Elimination Diet, Day 5; Rotation Diet, Day 3

Serves 4

50 g organic short wholegrain rice
1 litre mineral water
1 vanilla pod (optional)
1 to 2 tsp honey (optional)
1 tbsp safflower oil (optional)

Wash the grains and place in a saucepan with the water. Bring to the boil with the vanilla pod and simmer gently for 20 minutes to 1 hour. Cool slightly and then liquidise in a blender or in a baby mouli. Pour through a strainer and discard the pulp or use in recipes. Add the honey, and more water if necessary. Add the safflower oil when completely cool and keep refrigerated.

Cashew nut milk

Good for: Rotation Diet, Day 1

Serves 4

125 g cashew nuts
1 litre water
1 tbsp barley malt (optional)

Grind the cashew nuts in a liquidiser to a fine powder. Add some of the water and all of the barley malt and liquidise until smooth, gradually adding the remaining water. Keep chilled.

Almond milk

Good for: Preliminary Diet

Serves 4

125 g blanched almonds
1 litre mineral water
1 to 2 tsp honey
pinch of cinnamon

Liquidise the almonds and some of the water for a good minute, until the mixture is very smooth. Add the honey, cinnamon and remaining water, strain and serve. Cashew nuts may also be used.

Walnut, pecan nut and brazil nut milks can all be made in the same way.

Sunflower and sesame seed milk

Good for: Preliminary Diet

Serves 4

75 g organic sunflower seeds
25 g sesame seeds
500 ml mineral water
50 g organic dried dates

Rinse the seeds and liquidise with some of the water. When smooth, add the dates and the remaining water, blend again and serve. The fruit and seeds may be pre-soaked overnight.

Hot chocolate

Good for: Rotation Diet, Day 3

Serves 2

600 ml rice or soya milk
2 tsp cocoa powder
2 tsp honey

Bring the milk to the boil and stir in the cocoa powder and honey.

Soya milk

Good for: Elimination Diet, Day 13; Rotation Diet, Day 3

Serves 4

175 g organic soya beans

1 litre water

1 vanilla pod

1 tbsp safflower oil

1 to 2 tsp honey

Soak and sprout the soya beans for 4 to 5 days, rinsing twice a day. Place in a saucepan with the water and vanilla pod. Bring to the boil and then simmer gently until tender. Remove the vanilla pod and liquidise. Pour through a strainer and add the oil and honey to taste and extra water if necessary. Grape juice can also be used as a sweetener.

Pre-cooked soya flour may be used instead of beans and the ingredients liquidised together.

Honey egg nog

Good for: Rotation Diet, Day 3

Serves 2

600 ml rice milk (see page 234)

2 tsps honey

1 large free-range egg

pinch of nutmeg

Beat together the milk, honey and egg and sprinkle with nutmeg. 1 tbsp of carob powder can be added.

Carrot and cashew nut spread

Good for: Rotation Diet, Day 1

Serves 4

125 g carrots, cooked and puréed

125 g cashew nuts, ground

1 tbsp fresh parsley, finely chopped

pinch of sea salt or 1 tsp barley miso

sesame oil (optional)

Mix together the ingredients, adding a little sesame oil if necessary.

Mushroom and tahini spread

Good for: Rotation Diet, Day 1

Serves 4

125 g mushrooms, sliced

1 tbsp sesame oil

2 tbsp tahini

1 tbsp lemon juice

1 tsp barley miso

1 tbsp fresh parsley, finely chopped

Cook the mushrooms in the sesame seed oil until soft. Liquidise to a purée and mix well with the remaining ingredients.

Brazil nut butter

Good for: Rotation Diet, Day 2

Serves 4

125 g Brazil nuts

virgin olive oil

Wash the nuts and leave to soak overnight. Rinse off the water and then liquidise, dropping the nuts one by one onto the rotary blades. Add a little virgin olive oil to make a smooth paste. Eat immediately or freeze.

Hemp seed butter

Good for: Rotation Diet, Day 2

Serves 4

125 g hemp seeds

virgin olive oil

sea salt

Follow the recipe for Brazil nut butter but soak the hemp seeds for 48 hours before liquidising. The seeds may be lightly toasted using a dry frying pan and removing from the heat the moment they begin to pop.

Almond and sunflower seed butters

Good for: Rotation Diet, Day 3

Serves 4

Pre-soak the almonds or sunflower seeds over night. Rinse and then liquidise, dropping a few nuts or seeds at a time, onto the rotary blades. Add a pinch of salt to taste and a little of the corresponding cold pressed oil to make a paste. Use the same day or freeze.

Nut and seed butters

Good for: Preliminary Diet

Serves 4

Use any type of raw nut (except peanuts) or seed (pre-soaking overnight will make them sweeter and more digestible) and follow the method for almond and sunflower seed butters.

Hazelnut, walnut or pecan nut butter

Good for: Rotation Diet, Day 4

Serves 4

125 g hazelnuts

125 g walnuts or pecan nuts

1 tbsp walnut oil

sea salt

Use raw nuts and pre-soak if you wish. Grind in a liquidiser, dropping a few nuts at a time onto the rotary blades. Add a pinch of salt to taste and a little of the corresponding nut oil to make a paste. Spoon into a screw top jar and store in the refrigerator.

Hedgerow jam

Good for: Preliminary Diet

Makes approximately 6 x 200 g pots

675 g blackberries

225 g elderberries

225 g rose hips

125 g sloes

500 ml mineral water

250 ml pear juice

2 tbsp arrowroot or tapioca flour

Wash the fruit thoroughly and then stew in the water until soft. Pour through a sieve, stir in the pear juice to sweeten and thicken with arrowroot or tapioca flour. Keep refrigerated or freeze in small portions.

chapter 7 the next step

You can also help your body to recover by strengthening your immune system. A strong immune system will be able to fight off viruses, bacteria and other organisms and protect you from radiation, chemical pollution and all other toxic and poisonous substances far more effectively. This in turn will give your body more of a chance to re-balance, thus making any reactions less and less severe.

Deficiencies in vitamins or minerals can have a debilitating effect on the immune system, so it is important to eat good, nourishing food. Additional food supplements may also be necessary, especially when many foods need to be eliminated or when the nutrients in the foods are not being absorbed properly, which is often the case with allergy sufferers. However, it would be wise to consult a health practitioner before embarking on a programme so you do not waste money buying supplements of poor quality or ones that may cause adverse reactions. He or she will also be able to advise you on quantities. Here are some supplements that may be prescribed and prove to be useful:

Digestive enzymes
These can help break down undigested food components such as proteins. They consist of hydrochloric acid and pepsin, normally present in the stomach, and pancreatic enzymes normally present in the duodenum and small intestines. An alternative is to eat more raw food as the enzymes in the food will not have been destroyed by cooking.

Probiotics

These are a way of re-colonising good bacteria that may have been destroyed by drugs or poor diet. If harmful bacteria are allowed to take over, it can lead to conditions such as candidiasis. However, care needs to be taken in choosing a good quality supplement that contains Lactobacillus acidophilus and Bifidobacterium, either separately or together. Capsules should be bought in vacuum-sealed bottles and, once opened, kept in the refrigerator.

Soluble fibre

This helps to speed up the transport of food through the intestines. The longer poorly digested food stays in the gut, the more likely it is to cause problems. Fibre also helps to clean the walls of the intestines. The best sources are oat bran, rice bran, pectin and physillium husks.

Essential fatty acids (EFAs)

These are vital for the immune system, for the health and protection of the gastro-intestinal mucosa and the cell membranes throughout the body. The essential fatty acids are omega-3 (alpha linolenic acid) and omega-6 (linoleic acid). Flax seed oil is one of the best and richest sources of omega 3. This is also present in soya bean, walnut and wheat germ oils. Omega-6 EFAs are found in sesame seed oil, safflower, sunflower, corn and evening primrose oil. These oils should be unrefined and cold pressed and kept refrigerated once opened as oils can become rancid quite quickly and in this state they can affect the body adversely. Deficiency can result in stunted growth, hair loss, varicose veins, brittle nails, sexual immaturity, nervousness and skin disorders – especially eczema and dandruff.

Multi-minerals and vitamins

These may be necessary as it is increasingly difficult to obtain all the necessary amounts from foods alone.

Antioxidants

These include vitamins A,C,E; selenium, zinc, L-Cysteine and L-Glutathione. Apart from being important nutrients, these vitamins and minerals protect cells against harmful free radicals. A free radical is an atom or molecule with an unpaired electron. It can be extremely damaging because it attempts to pair its free electron with an electron from neighbouring molecules and can then set up a chain reaction causing damage to further cells. This 'latching on' process is called oxidation and can 'rust' the body almost as it does metal. Free radicals form because people are being exposed to thousands of substances, alien to the human body, such as atmospheric pollution, radiation, pesticides, additives, tobacco, alcohol, hard physical exercise, and many forms of medicines. Unsaturated fats, which are found naturally in cell membranes are particularly susceptible to free radical damage. The cell walls then become vulnerable to cancer, arteriosclerosis, arthritis, premature ageing and other diseases.

Vitamin C

This also has natural anti-inflammatory properties and it is important for iron absorption and in the production of collagen, a protein necessary for the formation of connective tissue in the skin, ligaments and bones. It also helps to control blood cholesterol levels and is an anti-stress factor. Deficiency may show itself in swollen gums, weakened enamel or dentine, sore joints, fatigue, lowered resistance to infection, nosebleeds, slow healing of wounds and poor complexion.

Ginkgo biloba

This is a herb which is also a powerful antioxidant and a useful protector for the intestinal mucosa. It improves the blood circulation in the hands, legs, feet and in the brain, thus improving memory and concentration.

The B vitamins

These are a group of vitamins that are essential for the release of energy from food and vital for the metabolism of proteins and fats. They help maintain a good circulation and healthy skin, hair and eyes. They contribute to the functioning of the brain and nervous system, to maintaining the correct balance of hormones in the body and to increasing one's ability to deal with stress.

Magnesium

This is needed for the metabolism of carbohydrates to release energy, for nerve impulse transmission and brain function and for normal muscle function including that of the heart. Symptoms of deficiency may include apprehensiveness, muscle twitches, tremors, confusion and forgetfulness, sleeplessness, the formation of clots in the heart and brain and may contribute to calcium deposits in the kidneys, blood vessels and heart. Our soil and hence the vegetable levels are low, so most of us could do with extra.

Iodine

This aids in the development and functioning of the thyroid gland, being a chief constituent of thyroxin, a principle hormone, and is particularly important for children and the elderly. Iodine plays an important role in regulating the body's production of energy, and it stimulates the rate of metabolism, helping the body to burn off excess fat. Mentality, speech and the condition of the hair, nails and skin and teeth are dependent upon a well functioning thyroid gland. Iodine is necessary for neutralising certain toxic substances and for protecting the body from the harmful effects of radiation. It is found in seaweed or can be taken in the form of kelp powder or tablets. Some kelp tablets contain milk powder, whey or lactose.

Zinc

This is necessary for the production of a vast number of enzymes and hormones present in the body. This is also a mineral, which has become very depleted in the soil. Stretch marks in the skin and white spots on the nails can be a sign of zinc deficiency. It may also produce an increase in fatigue, susceptibility to infection and a decrease in mental alertness.

Other ways of strengthening the immune system

In addition to diet and nutrition, we need to look at other aspects of our lives in order to strengthen our immune system and receive the benefits of good health. This includes taking sufficient exercise, fresh air and sunlight, our ability to relax, looking at our posture and breathing habits and above all, the quality of our thoughts.

We owe it to ourselves to be well. If we are well we have energy, vitality, and are a joy to be with. Health also gives us the ability to work and achieve our aims in life. Perhaps we think that by ignoring

---

Case study

Mary aged 49, was bothered by a lot of symptoms. She was overweight, had itching skin, tingling in her legs, weeping eyes, sensitivity to bright lights, hot flushes, palpitations, water retention, bloating, thrush, backache, pain in her muscles and joints, poor sleep, tension, anxiety, forgetfulness, difficulty in making decisions, aggressiveness, hyperactivity, constantly snacking, craving particular foods and little desire for sex. Mary found a nutritionist who considered that many symptoms might decrease if she changed her diet. Mary was found to be reacting to several foods: all dairy produce, potatoes, tomatoes, tea, peanuts as well as all pesticides on fruit and vegetables. After four months of avoiding these foods and eating organically produced fruit and vegetables, most of the symptoms had disappeared. Her head and eyes felt clearer than they had for years, her mood swings became a thing of the past and her crippling backache and other pains vanished. However, she still felt some anxiety. The hot flushes continued as did the tingling in her legs and she still felt overweight. Her practitioner then suggested she take a vitamin and mineral test to see how many deficiencies she had. It was discovered that Mary needed magnesium supplements, also zinc, selenium, iron and Vitamins C, B1, B2, B3 and B5. Her weight now is rapidly reducing, tingling in her legs does not occur, she is much less anxious and the hot flushes have almost disappeared. After years of misery, Mary is discovering what it is like to feel well again.

Philip developed hay fever at the age of two and was not a strong child. Constant infections kept him away from school. At twelve he developed severe depression, migraine symptoms, became very thin, occasionally hallucinated and eventually was not well enough to go to school at all. Philip was very ill for six years, but he then heard about elimination diets and food rotation. After the first week of eliminating the foods that he was reacting to, he was running about laughing and wanting to study. The headaches stopped and in the next two weeks all his various medicines were stopped. It took some time to regain good health, but Philip knew he was on the right track and he persisted. He persisted through a university course, cooking his own food and keeping to the principles of food rotation. He went backpacking across Canada, again carrying the special foods and finding places to cook. He then took some postgraduate courses and settled into a job. Careful maintenance of a rotation diet has made all this possible as well as homeopathic and radionic treatments. Philip has travelled across America, visited several European countries and travelled a lot in the United Kingdom. He has not let his diet prevent any of this.

problems, they will go away. However, we all know how much easier it is if we nip things in the bud. Take a dandelion growing out of place in a herbaceous border. When it first shows a couple of leaves it only takes a finger and thumb to remove it; leave it and the roots grow deeper until a garden spade and a surgical operation is needed to remove it, damaging surrounding flowers and plants in the procedure. We need to take heed of our own early warning signs.

It is now widely accepted that what we eat and how we prepare and cook our food can have an enormous effect on our health. You will have seen how one bite of a sandwich, or one sip of a drink can affect your entire body, both physically and mentally. But you also will have seen how to use food to your benefit. The choice is now up to you. Advances in transport and food distribution have brought an increasing abundance and array of fruits, vegetables and all kinds of different foods to our shops. So go out and experiment; say goodbye to the foods that can cause you problems – the 'convenience' foods full of additives, wheat, corn and dairy products, the fizzy drinks full of sugar, the chocolate and the potato chips. Instead, let your innate wisdom guide you to the right foods for you.

Working with the Elimination and Rotation Diets can be a valuable way of getting back to knowing yourself; knowing what your body needs and gradually becoming more 'in tune' with yourself and therefore with everything else in your life.

Appendix

Foods containing wheat:
wheat flour
wheat bran
wheatmeal
wheat-based crispbreads
wheat biscuits
wheat breakfast cereals (All-bran Weetabix, puffed wheat, muesli)
modified starch
baking powder
thickeners and binders
bakery products
some pumpernickel bread
cakes and cake mixes
batter mixes
spaghetti
macaroni and other pasta
pastry
mustard

also check the ingredients of the following:
Baked beans
chocolate and other sweets
cocoa
instant coffee
imitation cream
custard
instant puddings
spreads and pastes
some other flours e.g. rice flour
bean flours
buckwheat pasta
rye bread
sausages
beefburgers
hamburgers
corned beef
salami
luncheon meat
pâtés

foods coated in breadcrumbs or batter
canned soups
sauces –
• oxo cubes
• gravy
• white sauce
• Soya sauce
chutneys
alcoholic drinks –
• whisky
• most gins
• lager
• ale
• beer
• some wines
vitamin and mineral tablets

Foods containing milk and dairy products:
Cow's, goat's and sheep's milk
condensed, dried, evaporated, skimmed and powdered forms
butter
buttermilk
cream
cheese including dishes cooked with cheese
whey
lactose
casinates
margarines (check whey on labels)
yoghurts
custards
biscuits
cakes
ice-cream
foods cooked in batter
soups
sauces

sausages
prepared meats
most packets of convenience foods
some vitamin and mineral tablets

NB: Homoeopathic remedies can be obtained in a liquid form free from sac lac. Doctors can contact manufacturers to find pain relieving medicines which are milk free. Most tablets contain lactose.

Foods and products containing corn:
Adhesives
envelopes
stamps
stickers
lining of cans for vegetables
lining of paper plates and dishes
toothpaste
talcum powders
laundry starch
aspirin and other tablets
cough syrups
cornflower
sweetcorn
popcorn
biscuits
candies
instant coffee and tea
custard
instant whip puddings
ice cream
cornflakes
ales, beers, whisky and some wines
fizzy drinks
batters for frying
corn or maize oil
margarines containing maize oil
peanut butter
salad dressings
bleached white flour
powdered sugar

jam
milk in paper carton
beans and peas from cans
some brands of crisps
corn snacks
tortillas
gravy mixes and cubes
sausages
bacon
cured and tenderised ham
creamed soups
stuffing
glucose syrup and glucose in jams
mono sodium glutamate (Chinese foods)
distilled vinegar
Soya sauce
tomato sauce
salt shakers in cafes
pie fillings
fruit juices
canned and frozen fruits
Soya bean milks
boiled sweets
chewing gum
Vitamin C is derived from corn

Foods containing eggs:
Buns
croissants
Danish pastries
biscuits
cakes
flans
pastries and pies
salad dressings and salad cream
mayonnaise
some prepared salads
custard powder
ice-creams
lemon curd
instant whips and processed cream preparations
egg white in meringues

macaroons
marshmallows
sorbets
consommé soups
frostings and royal icings
Many vaccines are grown on egg and
    may cause reactions
batter mixes made with egg
quiches
fish cakes
egg pasta
enriched alcoholic drinks (egg-nogs)

Foods containing yeast:
Breads
some biscuits
crispbreads
cakes and cake mixes
flour enriched with vitamins from
    yeast
food coated in bread crumbs
some milk powders are fortified with
    vitamins from yeast (B vitamins)
mushrooms
truffles
cheese of all kinds
buttermilk and cottage cheese
vinegar and all convenience foods
    containing vinegar
gravy browning and similar extracts.
yeast/beef extracts
stock cubes
Fermented drinks –
• whisky
• gin
• wine
• brandy
• rum
• vodka
• beer etc.
Malted products –
• cereals
• sweets and chocolates
• milk drinks which have been
    malted

Citrus fruit juice (only home
    squeezed are yeast free)
Many B vitamins products are
    derived from yeast

Foods containing sugar:
Most alcoholic drinks
bakery products except stoneground
    wholemeal bread
instant coffee and tea
drinking chocolate
malted milk drinks
milk shakes
soft drinks and low calorie drinks
fruit juices and squashes except pure
    fruit juices
most breakfast cereals
most pre-cooked oven-ready foods
milk products –
• baby milks
• cream
• whipped cream
• ice cream
• processed cheeses
• some fruit yoghurts
all desserts
many frozen and packages foods
many jams
some honey may have sucrose
    added to it
sauces e.g. tomato sauce
Soya and other oriental sauces
mayonnaise
relishes
all sweets and candies
all tinned vegetables
fruits
soups
sauces
desserts are likely to contain sugar

Useful addresses

Association of Natural Medicine
27 Braintree Road, Witham,
Essex CM8 2DD.

British Complementary Medicine Association
Exmoor St. London W10 6DZ.

British Holistic Medical Association Trust
House, Royal Shrewsbury Hospital South,
Shrewsbury SY3 8XF.

Council for Complementary and Alternative Medicine
179 Gloucester Place,
London NW1 6DX.

Institute for Complementary Medicine
PO Box 194, London SE16 1QZ.

Natural Medicines Society
Edith Lewis House, Ikeston, Derbyshire.

Research Council for Complementary Medicine
60 Great Ormond Street,
London WC1N 3JF.

Society for the Promotion of Nutritional Therapy (SPNT)
PO Box 47, Heathfield,
East Sussex TN21 8ZX.

The Institute for Optimum Nutrition
Blades Court, Deodar Road
London SW15 2NU.

The Dr Lawrence Plaskett Nutritional Medicine College
23 Chapel Street, Camelford,
Cornwall PL32 9PJ.

Action Against Allergy
43 The Downs, London SW20.

Irish Allergy Association
PO Box 1067, Churchtown, Dublin.

Hyperactive Children's Support Group
71 Whyke Lane, Chichester,
West Sussex PO19 2LD.

Action for ME
PO Box 1302, Wells, Somerset BA5 2WE.

Foresight
The Old Vicarage, Witley, Godalming,
Surrey GU8 5PN.

The Radionic & Radiestheisic Organisation
Maperton Stud, Maperton, Wincanton,
Somerset BA9 8EH.

The General Council and Register of Naturopaths
Goswell House, 2 Goswell Road, Street,
Somerset BA16 0JG.

The Council for Acupuncture
179 Gloucester Place NW1 6DX.

Dr. Edward Bach Foundation
Mount Vermon, Sotwell,
Wallington OX10 0PZ.

The International Federation of Aromatherapists
Stamford House, 2–4 Chiswick High Road,
London W4 1TH.

The Colonic International Association
16 Englands Lane, London NW3 3TG.

The National Federation of Spiritual Healers
Old Manor Farm Studio, Church Street,
Sunbury-on-Thames, Middlesex TW16 6RG.

British Chiropractic Association
Equity House, 29 Whitley Street
Reading RG2 0EG.

McTimoney Chiropractic Association
21 High Street, Eynsham Oxon OX8 1HE.

Osteopathic Information Service
PO Box 2074, Reading, Berks RG1 4YR.

The General Council and Register of Naturopaths
6 Netherall Gardens, London NW3.

The Association of Systematic Kinesiology
39 Browns Road, Surbiton,
Surrey KT5 8ST.

Association of Reflexology
27 Old Gloucester Street,
London WC1N 3XX.

British Association for Counselling
1 Regent Place, Rugby CV21 2PJ.

The Radionic Association
Baerlein House, Goose Green, Deddington,
Oxon OX15 0SZ.

National Institute of Medical Herbalists
56 Longbrook St, Exeter, Devon EX4 6AH.

British Homoeopathic Association
27a Devonshire St, London W1N 1RJ.

The Centre for the Study of Complementary Medicine
51 Bedford Place, Southampton,
Hants SO1 2DG.

St. Braivels Centre for Child Development
Dixton Road, Monmouth, Gwent NP5 3PR.

Food products

Newtown Farm
South Gorley, Fordingbridge, Hants.
(organic meat)

Swaddles Green Farm
Hare Lane, Buckland St Mary, Chard,
Somerset TA20 3JR.
(organic meat, mail order)

Trenchman's
The Old Dairy, Compton Park, Sherborne,
Dorset. (wild game, wild boar, frozen fish
etc. mail order)

Allergy Care (incorporating Foodwatch International Ltd)
9 Corporation Street, Taunton,
Somerset TA1 4AJ. (Mail order wholefoods)

Wild Oats (Mail order)
210 Westbourne Grove,
London W11 2RH. (wholefoods)

Freshland (Mail order)
196 Old Street London EC1V 9FR.
(wholefoods)

Savant Distribution Ltd.
7 Wayland Croft, Adel, Leeds LS16 8LA.
(organic cold pressed oils)

The House of Hemp
1st Floor, 31–39 Redchurch Street,
Shoreditch, London E2 7DJ.

Higher Nature
The Nutritional Centre, Burwash Common,
East Sussex TN19 7LX. (mail order
nutritional supplements)

Overseas addresses
Allergy Foundation of America
801 Second Avenue, New York NY 10017.

American Academy of Advancement in Medicine (ACAM)
23121 Verdugo Drive, #204 Laguna Hills,
CA 92653.
Tel: (714) 583-7666

American Academy of Environmental Medicine
Prairie Village, Kansas.
Tel: (913) 642-6062

AMR'TA – Alchemical Medicine and Teaching Association
P.O. Box 634, Beaverton, OR 97075-0634.
Tel: (503) 644-7840
E-mail: amrta@amrta.org

International Academy of Nutrition and Preventative Medicine
P.O. Box 5832, Lincoln NE 68505.
Tel: (402) 467-2716.

AIA Allergy Information Association
3 Powburn Place, Weston, Ontario, Canada.

Allergy Association Australia
P.O. Box 298, Ringwood,
Victoria 3134, Austalia.

Allergy Recognition and Management
P.O. Box 2, Sandy Bay, Tasmania 7005.

Allergy Awareness Association
P.O. Box 120701, Penrose,
Auckland 6, New Zealand.

Further reading

Erasmus, Udo, *Fats that Heal, Fats that Kill*, Alive Books, Canada.

Davies, Gwynne, *Overcoming Food Allergies*, Ashgrove.

Mackarness, R. *Not all in the Mind*, Pan.

Mackarness, R. *Chemical Victims*, Pan.

Randolph, T & Moss, R. *Allergies: Your Hidden Enemy*. Turnstone.

Needes, R. *You Don't Have To Feel Unwell*. Gateway.

Dr. S. Davies and Dr. A. Stewart. *Nutritional Medicine*. Pan Books.

Dr. Mansfield, P & Dr. Munro, J. *Chemical Children*. Century Paperbacks.

Schause, A. *Diet, Crime & Delinquency*, Parker House (USA)

Bloomfield, B. *The Mystique of Healing*. Skilton & Shaw.

Dr. Lewith, G, Dr. Kenyon, J & Dr Dowson, D. *Allergy and Intolerance*. Merlin Press.

Dr. Brostoff, J & Gamlin, L. *Food allergy and Intolerance*. Bloomsbury.

Dr. Dong, *New Hope for the Arthritic*, Granada Press.

Mental and Elemental Nutrients, Brain Bio Centre, Princetown, New Jersey, USA.

Dr. Galland, L, Allergy *Prevention for Kids*. Bloomsbury.

Rapp, Doris J. *Allergies and the Hyperactive Child*. Sterling Publishing, New York.

Budd, Martin, *Low Blood Sugar*, Thorsons.

Dr Joneja, Janice, M.D., *Dietary Management of Food Allergies and Intolerances*

Index

You may also be interested in the following Vermilion titles:

Dr Atkins New Diet Revolution by Dr Robert Atkins

Eat Fat, Get Thin! by Barry Groves

The Body Clock Diet by Dr Sidney MacDonald Baker & Karen Baar

The Gut Reaction Eating Plan by Gudrun Jonsson

The IBS Starch-Free Diet by Carol Sinclair

The New 5 Day Miracle Diet by Adele Puhn

The New High Protein Diet by Professor Charles Clark

To obtain a copy, simply telephone TBS Direct on 01206 255800